Ovulation Induction

REPRODUCTIVE MEDICINE AND ASSISTED REPRODUCTIVE TECHNIQUES SERIES

David Gardner
University of Melbourne, Australia

Zeev Shoham
Kaplan Hospital, Rehovot, Israel

Kay Elder, Jacques Cohen
Human Preimplantation Embryo Selection, ISBN: 9780415399739

John D Aplin, Asgerally T Fazleabas, Stanley R Glasser, Linda C Giudice
The Endometrium, Second Edition, ISBN: 9780415385831

Nick Macklon, Ian Greer, Eric Steegers
Textbook of Periconceptional Medicine, ISBN: 9780415458924

Andrea Borini, Giovanni Coticchio
Preservation of Human Oocytes, ISBN: 9780415476799

Steven R Bayer, Michael M Alper, Alan S Penzias
The Boston IVF Handbook of Infertility, Third Edition, ISBN: 9781841848105

Ben Cohlen, Willem Ombelet
Intra-Uterine Insemination: Evidence Based Guidelines for Daily Practice,
ISBN: 9781841849881

Adam H. Balen
Infertility in Practice, Fourth Edition, ISBN: 9781841848495

Nick Macklon
IVF in the Medically Complicated Patient, Second Edition:
A Guide to Management, ISBN: 9781482206692

Michael Tucker, Juergen Liebermann
Vitrification in Assisted Reproduction, ISBN: 9780415408820

Ben J Cohlen, Evert J P van Santbrink, Joop S E Laven
Ovulation Induction: Evidence Based Guidelines for Daily Practice,
ISBN: 9781498704076

Ovulation Induction
Evidence Based Guidelines for Daily Practice

Edited by

Ben J. Cohlen, M.D., Ph.D.
Isala Fertility Center
Zwolle, The Netherlands

Evert J. P. van Santbrink, M.D., Ph.D.
Department of Reproductive Medicine, Diaconessenhuis Voorburg
Reinier de Graafgroep
Voorburg, The Netherlands

Joop S. E. Laven, M.D., Ph.D.
Division of Reproductive Medicine, Department of Obstetrics
and Gynecology, Erasmus Medical Center
Rotterdam, The Netherlands

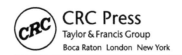

CRC Press
Taylor & Francis Group
Boca Raton London New York

CRC Press is an imprint of the
Taylor & Francis Group, **an informa** business

CRC Press
Taylor & Francis Group
6000 Broken Sound Parkway NW, Suite 300
Boca Raton, FL 33487-2742

© 2017 by Taylor & Francis Group, LLC
CRC Press is an imprint of Taylor & Francis Group, an Informa business

No claim to original U.S. Government works

Printed on acid-free paper
Version Date: 20160311

International Standard Book Number-13: 978-1-4987-0407-6 (Paperback)

Library of Congress Cataloging-in-Publication Data

Names: Cohlen, Ben, 1963- , editor. | Santbrink, Evert van, editor. | Laven, Joop, editor.
Title: Ovulation induction : evidence based guidelines for daily practice / editors, Ben J. Cohlen, Evert van Santbrink, and Joop Laven.
Other titles: Ovulation induction (Cohlen) | Reproductive medicine & assisted reproductive techniques series.
Description: Boca Raton : Taylor & Francis, 2017. | Series: Reproductive medicine and assisted reproductive techniques series | Includes bibliographical references and index.
Identifiers: LCCN 2016011402 | ISBN 9781498704076 (pbk. : alk. paper)
Subjects: | MESH: Ovulation Induction--methods | Anovulation--etiology | Gonadotropins--therapeutic use
Classification: LCC RG137.3 | NLM WP 540 | DDC 618.1/84--dc23
LC record available at http://lccn.loc.gov/2016011402

Visit the Taylor & Francis Web site at
http://www.taylorandfrancis.com

and the CRC Press Web site at
http://www.crcpress.com

Contents

Foreword

Today there is less and less emphasis on the elucidation of possible causes of infertility, and, consequently, fertility specialists and patients often rush to empirical interventions. It is therefore good to see that the current book is dedicated fully to one of the most common causes of infertility (anovulation) and its causal treatment. Ovarian dysfunction can be recognized easily because it results in the deviation of the normal pattern of regular menstrual bleeding. Oligo- or amenorrhea is thought to occur in approximately 10% to 15% of infertile couples, and the understanding of relevant causal factors is essential for safe and effective treatment. Moreover, general health issues may coincide with ovarian dysfunction.

The classification of anovulatory infertility has been essentially unaltered for more than half a century since just after the first radio-immunoassays became available for assessing steroid serum concentrations in clinical practice. This was way before clinical investigators became aware of the evidence-based methods in research and clinical implementation. Even today, the simple measurement of hormone concentrations in the peripheral circulation can fairly accurately delineate whether anovulation is primarily due to hypothalamic–pituitary dysfunction, abnormalities residing within the ovary itself, or a loosely defined "hormone dysbalance." By far the most common diagnosis associated with anovulatory infertility is the notoriously heterogeneous condition referred to as polycystic ovary syndrome.

Ovarian stimulation represents a fundamental component of many current infertility treatments. The term "ovulation induction" should be restricted to the medical treatment of anovulation with the aim to achieve single dominant follicle selection resulting in the release of a single oocyte and hopefully a singleton pregnancy. Compelling evidence demonstrated that this can now be performed safely by medication, minimal ovarian surgery, or a combination of both. When compounds for ovarian stimulation became available in the early '60s of the previous century (i.e., urinary gonadotrophins and the anti-estrogen clomiphene citrate), this approach was rapidly adopted for the large-scale treatment of anovulatory infertility. Ovulation induction has been successful in inducing ovulation and pregnancy right from the beginning. The aim of singleton follicle development and ovulation was often not achieved at the beginning, resulting in an unacceptably high multiple pregnancy rate up to 40%. With current strategies for ovulation induction and proper ovarian response monitoring, effective treatment is possible with cumulative singleton pregnancy rates described up to 80%–90%. The major risk associated with direct ovarian stimulation remains the rare but potentially dangerous ovarian hyperstimulation syndrome. Recent studies involving adequately powered randomized comparative trials helped to delineate most effective interventions, and novel compounds for ovulation induction, such as insulin-sensitizing agents and aromatase inhibitors, continue to be introduced.

More recently, ovarian stimulation is also used in the context of assisted reproduction, aiming to stimulate the development of multiple dominant follicles in normo-ovulatory women. Such an approach can be used for the empirical treatment of unexplained infertility or in combination with intrauterine insemination with the inherent risk of higher multiple pregnancy rates. In the great majority of cases, ovarian hyperstimulation is used in the context of in vitro fertilization (IVF), with which chances of multiple pregnancy can be reduced by diminishing the number of embryos transferred.

In case ovulation induction does not result in a pregnancy, the following treatment modality is usually IVF. Overall, clinical outcomes are good although complication rates may be increased, especially in women with PCOS.

Finally, we should be aware of the fact that a positive pregnancy test should not be considered the final end point of ovulation induction. Next to pregnancy complications associated with multiple pregnancies even singleton pregnancies can be at increased risk for complications, especially associated with increased or decreased body weight and its metabolic implications. Accordingly, more attention should be directed toward the prospective follow-up of pregnancy, perinatal outcomes, and future health of children.

This book summarizes the existing evidence in a comprehensive and practical way. After reading all chapters, we might conclude that future research in anovulation is still warranted, and many aspects, for instance genetics in PCO and WHO 3, seem exciting. There is still a need for randomized trials and evidence-based guidelines to offer couples optimal perspectives with minimal complications. This book might help colleagues in constructing these guidelines.

Bart C. J. M. Fauser, MD, PhD
Professor of Reproductive Medicine
Utrecht, The Netherlands

Evidence Evaluation

The levels of evidence used in the statements in this text are as follows:

1a	Systematic review and meta-analysis of randomized controlled trials
1b	At least one randomized controlled trial
2a	At least one well-designed, controlled study without randomization
2b	At least one other type of well-designed quasiexperimental study
3	Well-designed, nonexperimental descriptive studies, such as comparative studies, correlation studies, or case studies
4	Expert committee reports or opinions and/or clinical experience of respected authorities

The strength of evidence is graded as follows for the recommendations (guidelines) in this text:

A	Directly based on Level 1 evidence
B	Directly based on Level 2 evidence or extrapolated recommendation from Level 1 evidence
C	Directly based on Level 3 evidence or extrapolated recommendation from either Levels 1 or 2 evidence
D	Directly based on Level 4 evidence or extrapolated recommendation from either Levels 1, 2, or 3 evidence
GPP	Good practice point

Contributors

Saad Amer
Division of Medical Sciences and Graduate
    Entry Medicine
University of Nottingham
Royal Derby Hospital
Derby, United Kingdom

Miriam Baumgarten
Addenbrooke's Hospital
Cambridge University Hospitals
Cambridge, United Kingdom

Neriman Bayram
Zaans Medisch Centrum
Department of Obstetrics and Gynaecology
Zaandam, the Netherlands

Jacqueline Boyle
Monash Centre for Health Research and
    Implementation
School of Public Health and Preventive
    Medicine
Monash University
Clayton, Australia

Miriam Braakhekke
Department of Obstetrics and Gynecology
Center for Reproductive Medicine
Academic Medical Center
Amsterdam, the Netherlands

Frank J. M. Broekmans
Department of Reproductive Medicine
University Medical Center Utrecht
Utrecht, the Netherlands

Robert F. Casper
Department of Obstetrics and Gynecology
University of Toronto
and
The Lunenfeld-Tanenbaum Research Institute
and
TRIO Fertility
Toronto, Ontario, Canada
and
Insception-Lifebank Cord Blood Bank

Isabelle Cédrin-Durnerin
Reproductive Medicine Center
Jean-Verdier Hospital (Assistance Publique—
    Hôpitaux de Paris)
University Paris XIII
Paris, France

Sophie Christin-Maitre
Endocrine Unit
AP-HP Hôpital Saint-Antoine
Université Paris VI
and
INSERM U933
Hôpital Trousseau
Paris, France

Ben J. Cohlen
Isala Fertility Centre
Isala
Zwolle, the Netherlands

Annelien C. de Kat
Department of Reproductive Medicine
University Medical Center Utrecht
Utrecht, the Netherlands

Diane De Neubourg
Center for Reproductive Medicine
Antwerp University Hospital
Edegem, Belgium

Didier Dewailly
CHU Lille
Department of Endocrine Gynaecology and
    Reproductive Medicine
Hôpital Jeanne de Flandre
Centre Hospitalier de Lille
Lille, France

Héctor F. Escobar-Morreale
Department of Endocrinology and Nutrition
Hospital Universitario Ramon y Cajal
    and Universidad de Alcalá and Instituto Ramón
    y Cajal de Investigación Sanitaria (IRYCIS)
    and CIBER Diabetes y Enfermedades
    Metabólicas Asociadas (CIBERDEM)
Madrid, Spain

Panagiota Filippou
Homerton Fertility Centre
Homerton University Hospital
London, United Kingdom

Kathrin Fleischer
Division of Reproductive Medicine
Department of Obstetrics and Gynaecology
Radboud University Medical Centre
Nijmegen, the Netherlands

Camille Grysole
CHU Lille
Department of Endocrine Gynaecology and
    Reproductive Medicine
Hôpital Jeanne de Flandre
Centre Hospitalier de Lille
Lille, France

Roy Homburg
Homerton Fertility Centre
Homerton University Hospital
London, United Kingdom

Jean-Noël Hugues
Reproductive Medicine Center
Jean-Verdier Hospital (Assistance Publique—
    Hôpitaux de Paris)
University Paris XIII
Paris, France

Fahrettin Keleştimur
Department of Endocrinology and Metabolism
Erciyes University
School of Medicine
Kayseri, Turkey

Anat Hershko Klement
Division of Reproductive Sciences
Fran and Lawrence Bloomberg Department
    of Obstetrics and Gynecology
University of Toronto
The Lunenfeld-Tanenbaum Research Institute
Mount Sinai Hospital
and
TCART Fertility Partners
Toronto, Ontario, Canada

Walter Kuchenbecker
Fertility Center Isala
Isala Clinics
Zwolle, the Netherlands

Cornelis B. Lambalk
Division of Reproductive Medicine
Department of Obstetrics and Gynaecology
VU University Medical Centre
Amsterdam, the Netherlands

Joop S. E. Laven
Division of Reproductive Medicine
Department of Obstetrics and Gynaecology
Erasmus University Medical Centre
Rotterdam, the Netherlands

Richard S. Legro
Obstetrics and Gynecology
Pennsylvania State University College of Medicine
Hershey, Pennsylvania

Sharon V. Lie Fong
University Hospitals Leuven
Department of Gynaecology and Obstetrics
Leuven University Fertility Centre
Leuven, Belgium

Yvonne V. Louwers
Division of Reproductive Medicine
Reinier de Graaf Group
Voorburg, the Netherlands

Nick S. Macklon
Department of Obstetrics and Gynaecology
University of Southampton
Southampton, United Kingdom

and

Zealand University Hospital
University of Copenhagen
Copenhagen, Denmark

Marie Misso
Monash Centre for Health Research and
    Implementation
School of Public Health and Preventive Medicine
Monash University
Clayton, Australia

Ben W. Mol
Robinson Research Institute
School of Pediatrics and Reproductive Health
University of Adelaide
Adelaide, Australia

Lisa J. Moran
Monash Centre for Health Research and
    Implementation
School of Public Health and Preventive
    Medicine
Monash University
Clayton, Australia

and

Robinson Research Institute
Discipline of Obstetrics and Gynaecology
University of Adelaide
Adelaide, Australia

Alex F. Muller
Department of Internal Medicine
Diakonessenhuis Utrecht
Utrecht, The Netherlands

Marleen Nahuis
Spaarne Gasthuis
Haarlem, the Netherlands

Sebastian J. C. M. M. Neggers
Department of Medicine
Section Endocrinology
and
Pituitary Center Rotterdam
Erasmus University Medical Centre
Rotterdam, the Netherlands

Scott M. Nelson
Department of Reproductive and Maternal
    Medicine
University of Glasgow
Glasgow, Scotland

Renato Pasquali
Endocrinology Unit
Department of Medical and Surgical Sciences
University Alma Mater Studiorum of Bologna
S. Orsola-Malpighi Hospital
Bologna, Italy

Botros Rizk
Division of Reproductive Medicine and Infertility
Department of Obstetrics and Gynecology
University of South Alabama
Mobile, Alabama

Mili Saran
Consultant in Reproductive Medicine
Complete Fertility Centre
Southampton University Hospital
Southampton, United Kingdom

Jean-Pierre Siffroi
Université Paris VI
and
Cytogenetic and Molecular Genetic Unit
Hôpital Trousseau
Paris, France

Helena J. Teede
Monash Centre for Health Research and
    Implementation
School of Public Health and Preventive Medicine
Monash University
Clayton, Australia

Aart J. van der Lely
Department of Medicine
Section Endocrinology
and
Pituitary Center Rotterdam
Erasmus University Medical Centre
Rotterdam, the Netherlands

Evert J. P. van Santbrink
Division of Reproductive Medicine
Reinier de Graaf Group
Voorburg, the Netherlands

Madelon van Wely
Department of Obstetrics and Gynecology
Center for Reproductive Medicine
Academic Medical Center
Amsterdam, the Netherlands

1

Physiology of the Menstrual Cycle: Understanding the Principles of Ovarian Stimulation

Mili Saran and Nick S. Macklon

Introduction

Following the pioneering days of in vitro fertilization (IVF), ovarian stimulation became an integral part of assisted reproductive techniques (ARTs). Over the last three decades, ovarian stimulation protocols have undergone numerous refinements in an effort to optimize the follicular phase of ovarian stimulation and, increasingly, the resulting luteal phase, too.

Optimal use of ovarian stimulation protocols requires a clear understanding of the physiological regulation of the ovarian cycle and the precise aims of interventions designed to mimic or override it. Moreover, as the role of the endometrium as a determinant of treatment outcomes becomes clearer, an understanding of the relationship of the cyclical phases of endometrial development is important. This chapter therefore addresses the regulation of the ovarian cycle (follicular phase, triggering of ovulation, and luteal phase) and the endometrial cycle (proliferative phase, secretory phase, and menstrual phase).

Ovarian Cycle

The Follicular Phase

The initial growth of primordial follicles (also referred to as "primary" recruitment) is random, being independent of follicle-stimulating hormone (FSH). The regulation of early follicular development and atresia and the degree to which FSH influences this remains unclear (1). Studies in women with a mutated FSH beta subunit have shown follicular growth to occur up to the stage of secondary recruitment without the need for FSH. Factors such as TGF-alpha from theca cells, growth differentiation factor 9 (GDF), and bone morphogenetic protein 15 produced by the oocyte may limit the effects of FSH on granulosa cell differentiation and follicle development at this early stage (1). Throughout reproductive life, gonadotrophin-releasing hormone (GnRH) is released from the hypothalamus in a pulsatile manner and stimulates the synthesis and release of FSH and luteinizing hormone (LH) by the anterior pituitary gland.

In the non-conception cycle, due to the involution of the corpus luteum during the late luteal phase of the menstrual cycle, estradiol (E2), inhibin A, and progesterone (P) levels fall. These, in turn, cause increased slow pulse frequencies (<1 pulse per 2–3 hour) of GnRH secretion, inducing rising levels of FSH at the end of the luteal phase. Only those antral follicles that happen to be at a more advanced stage of maturation during the inter-cycle rise in FSH gain gonadotrophin dependence and continue to grow (2). This process is referred to as cyclic, gonadotropin-dependent, or "secondary" recruitment. The cohort size of healthy early antral follicles recruited during the luteo-follicular transition is around 10 per ovary, based on indirect observations. The theca cells of the maturing follicle develop LH receptors and synthesize androstenedione while the granulosa cells respond to FSH and synthesize aromatase enzyme, which, in turn, converts the androstenedione to estradiol (E2) (the two cell–two gonadotrophin theory) (3,4).

Inhibin B, secreted by the recently recruited cohort of follicles in response to FSH, rapidly rises immediately after the inter-cycle rise in FSH (2). This rise in inhibin B, along with the rising estradiol (E2) levels during the mid and late follicular phase, has negative feedback at the hypothalamic–pituitary axis causing a steady decrease in serum FSH levels. This secures the selection of a single dominant follicle, which becomes less dependent on FSH and continues to grow in a natural cycle. The remaining follicles from the recruited cohort cease to mature and undergo atresia through a process of apoptosis (Figures 1.1 and 1.2).

Decreasing follicular phase FSH levels (effectively restricting the time when FSH levels remain above the threshold, referred to as the FSH window) is crucial for selecting a single dominant follicle from the recruited cohort. The key role of FSH in stimulating preovulatory follicle growth has been demonstrated by the use of exogenous FSH to stimulate follicle growth up to the preovulatory stage in hypophysectomized women (1,4). Although granulosa cells from early antral follicles respond only to FSH, those from mature follicles (exhibiting receptors to both gonadotropins) are responsive to both FSH and LH. The maturing dominant follicle may become less dependent on FSH because of the ability to respond to LH (1).

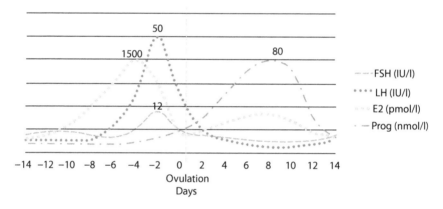

FIGURE 1.1 Graphic representation of variation in pituitary and ovarian hormonal levels during menstrual cycle (not to scale).

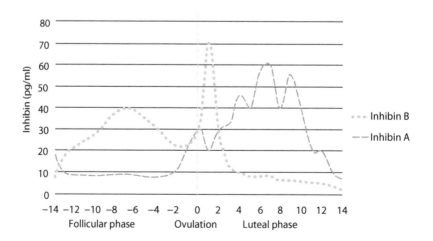

FIGURE 1.2 Graphic representation of inhibin A and B levels during menstrual cycle (not to scale) (2,3).

The LH Surge and the Luteal Phase

Rising levels of E2, produced by the granulosa cells of the preovulatory dominant follicle, cause the release of fast pulse frequencies (>1 pulse per hour) and high amplitude GnRH, favoring increased LH production (2). This causes a switch from a negative to positive feedback effect, resulting in a rapid rise in LH release and the so-called LH surge. The initial onset of the LH surge (not the peak level, which is reached 10–12 hours before ovulation) induces the ovulation about 34–36 hours later. The mean duration of the LH surge is 48 hours. Besides triggering ovulation, the LH surge induces the formation of the corpus luteum, for which an adequate amplitude and duration of LH surge is essential. The wall of the follicle collapses, and capillaries invade the developing corpus luteum probably under the influence of angiogenic and mitogenic factors. The differentiated granulosa cells in the corpus luteum will produce progesterone (P) in increasing amounts, E2, and inhibin A (1,2).

In some species, such as rodents, prolactin-like hormones play a principal role in the luteotropic process, and luteal regression involves a uterine signal such as prostaglandin F2 alpha (1). In contrast to this, in humans, LH is the principle hormone responsible for the following events. First, the mid-cycle surge of gonadotropins (notably, LH) stimulates the resumption of oocyte meiotic maturation; rupture of the dominant follicle, allowing the release of oocyte (ovulation), and corpus luteum formation (i.e., luteinization). Second, the pulsatile secretion of pituitary LH during the luteal phase of the menstrual cycle promotes the continued development and normal functional lifespan of the corpus luteum (1,2).

And finally, the exponential rise in circulating levels of the LH-like hormone, chorionic gonadotropin (CG), secreted by the implanting blastocyst and syncytiotrophoblast of the developing placenta, extends the functional lifespan of the corpus luteum in early pregnancy until luteal activities are assumed by the placenta, that is, at the luteal–placental shift (1,4).

Studies during the 1970s and 1980s and more recent experiments using GnRH antagonists and pure recombinant human LH or human CG (hCG) have strengthened the critical role of LH/CG in regulating primate luteal structure–function and is increasingly being applied in ovarian stimulation for IVF (1).

Although the maturing dominant follicle may be less sensitive to acute LH withdrawal at mid-cycle, a GnRH-induced LH surge of substantial length is required for ovulation and development of normal luteal function. What remains unclear is how duration and/or amplitude of the mid-cycle LH surge influences peri-ovulatory events. Initial monkey and human studies on GnRH-induced LH surges or administering exogenous LH/CG suggest that surges of lesser duration (<24 hours) and amplitude are sufficient to reinitiate oocyte meiosis and granulosa cell luteinization, but surges of greater duration (>24 hours) and amplitude improve oocyte recovery, fertilization, and corpus luteum development (1,2). Although the LH surge is believed to be the physiological signal for peri-ovulatory events, studies in rodents showed that a mid-cycle bolus of FSH can replace LH and elicit oocyte maturation, ovulation, and successful pregnancy (1). The clinical relevance of these physiological observations has recently been brought into sharper focus by the use of GnRHa agonists to induce a mid-cycle LH surge in IVF cycles. Although the short period of stimulation reduces the risk of developing ovarian hyperstimulation syndrome, it is clear that it may impact detrimentally on the luteal phase, compared with the use of hCG as a trigger, which remains bioactive for a longer period. These clinical issues are addressed elsewhere.

The LH-stimulated luteinization of granulosa cells around ovulation includes enhanced vascular endothelial growth factor (VEGF) production, which is likely essential for the angiogenic process within the corpus luteum. With regards to hCG, a mid-cycle bolus in ovarian stimulation cycles increased expression of the endogenous angiopoietin agonist, Ang-1, without altering that of the endogenous antagonist, Ang-2, in macaque granulosa cells. These factors control not only the development or maintenance of the vasculature in developing tissue beds, but also vascular integrity, maturity, and permeability (1). It has been proposed that overexpression, increased bioavailability, or a change in the ratio of angiogenic factors, notably VEGF-A, is a cause of ovarian hyperstimulation syndrome (OHSS), a serious side effect of ovarian stimulation characterized by intravascular volume loss and extravascular fluid accumulation. The early or late occurrence of OHSS in ovarian stimulation cycles has been linked to the ovulatory hCG bolus and endogenous CG production at pregnancy recognition, respectively (1,2).

The Endometrium

The basalis layer that remains after shedding of the more superficial endometrium at menstruation needs to regrow and differentiate (proliferative phase) under the E2 influence secreted by the growing follicles in the follicular phase of the ovarian cycle. The highest E2 response is in the glands via increased E2 receptor (ER) expression (4). First, there is an increase in the mitotic activity, and second, there is formation of a loose capillary network in the spiral vessels. After ovulation, the progesterone (P) produced by the corpus luteum causes the cessation of endometrial proliferation and initiates glandular secretion (secretory phase). The endometrial glands become tortuous and spiral vessels coiled. During the secretory phase, a short specific period of uterine receptivity toward embryonic implantation is designated as the "implantation window" (2,4). Available evidence based on experimental studies supports the discrete time in the cycle between 6 and 10 days after the LH surge that defines this window of implantation (1). Coinciding with this window, the expression of cell adhesion molecules such as integrins, under endocrine and paracrine control, may assist in the initial stages of implantation of the embryo. If conception and implantation occur, the developing blastocyst secretes human chorionic gonadotrophin (hCG), which, in turn, supports and maintains the corpus luteum until the developing placenta takes over steroidogenesis. Continued progesterone exposure also promotes local vasodilatation and uterine musculature quiescence by inducing nitric oxide synthesis in the decidua (1,4).

In the absence of implantation, luteolysis is initiated after 12 days, and P and inhibin A levels decrease, resulting in menstruation. As a result of a reduced negative feedback effect, GnRH pulse frequency will increase, and subsequently, pituitary FSH production will increase and, again, the inter-cycle will rise (2).

The major roles of E2 are for endometrial growth and for enabling P to act on the endometrial tissue—both stroma and glands. To accomplish these goals, E2 induces progesterone receptor (PR) expression and promotes cellular proliferation in the tissue directly through its cognate receptors and indirectly by induction of growth factors that act as autocrine and/or paracrine modulators (1).

With regard to PR, peak expression in human endometrium induced by E2 is at the time of ovulation. PR is most prominent in the glandular epithelium in the proliferative phase. In contrast, stromal cells have high levels of PR in the follicular phase and throughout the luteal phase. Timely downregulation of epithelial PR coincides with the opening of the window of implantation and uterine receptivity for embryonic implantation, and histological delay of the endometrium (a clinically abnormal state) is associated with a failure of such PR downregulation (1).

Recent Advances

The pulsatile release of GnRH is key to starting the menstrual cycle at puberty. Any disruption in the pulse frequency will give rise to reproductive dysfunction. Kisspeptin and neurokinin B (NKB), neuropeptides secreted by the same neuronal population in the ventral hypothalamus, have recently emerged as crucial central regulators of GnRH and hence gonadotropin secretion. Patients with mutations resulting in loss of signaling by either of these neuroendocrine peptides fail to attain puberty, but the mechanisms mediating this remain unclear (5).

Recent animal and human studies have shown that continuous kisspeptin infusion restores gonadotropin pulsatility in patients with loss of function mutations in NKB or its receptor, indicating that kisspeptin on its own is sufficient to stimulate pulsatile GnRH secretion (Figures 1.3 and 1.4) (5,6). The studies also suggest that NKB action is proximal to kisspeptin in the reproductive neuroendocrine cascade regulating GnRH secretion and may act as an autocrine modulator of kisspeptin secretion. The ability of continuous kisspeptin infusion to induce pulsatile gonadotropin secretion further indicates that GnRH neurons are able to set up pulsatile secretion in the absence of pulsatile exogenous kisspeptin (5,6).

These findings suggest a potential future role of kisspeptin and NKB in treating dysfunctions of the reproductive system and hormone-dependent diseases (5,6).

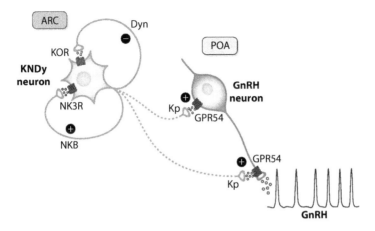

FIGURE 1.3 Suggested model for the role of kisspeptin neurons (KNDy) expressing both neurokinin B (NKB) and dynorphin A (Dyn) neurons in the control of pulsatile GnRH secretion. A schematic model for the likely roles of NKB and Dyn as co-transmitters and possible regulators of the secretory activity of Kiss1 neurons, located at the arcuate nuclei (ARC) as a major driving signal for GnRH pulsatile release by GnRH neurons sited in the preoptic area (POA). (From http://physrev .physiology.org/content/92/3/1235, with permission.)

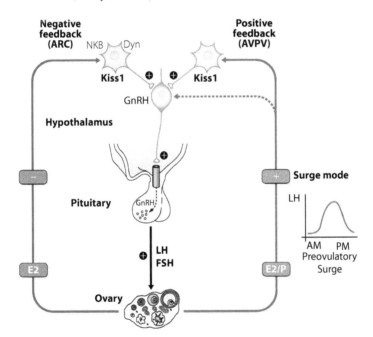

FIGURE 1.4 Differential regulation and actions of ARC versus anteroventral peri-ventricular nucleus (AVPV) Kiss1 neurons in the control of GnRH in rodents. A schematic illustration of the roles of Kiss1 neurons in the ARC and AVPV in mediating the negative and positive feedback effects of ovarian sex steroids on GnRH and gonadotropin secretion as suggested on the basis of female rodent data. (From http://physrev.physiology.org/content/92/3/1235, with permission.)

Conclusion

This chapter outlines the endocrine and paracrine control of the ovarian and concurrent menstrual cycles in the light of available evidence. This acknowledges the complex molecular interactions, and how this could be implied in the context of ART as well as looking into the scope of further research, where the mechanisms are still less clearly understood.

TABLE 1.1

Level of Evidence of Statements

Statement	Level of Evidence
The initial growth of primordial follicles (also referred to as primary recruitment) is random, being independent of FSH. The cohort size of healthy early antral follicles recruited during the luteo-follicular transition is around 10 per ovary.	3
Inhibin A, secreted by maturing follicle and corpus luteum, has a direct endocrine role in the negative feedback on pituitary FSH production.	2b
Although the LH surge is believed to be the physiological signal for peri-ovulatory events, a mid-cycle bolus of FSH can replace LH and elicit oocyte maturation, ovulation, early luteinization of granulosa cells, and successful pregnancy.	2b
The major roles of E2 on uterine endometrium are for endometrial growth and for enabling P to act on the tissue.	2b
Kisspeptin and neurokinin B (NKB), neuropeptides secreted by the same neuronal population in the ventral hypothalamus, have emerged recently as critical central regulators of GnRH and thus gonadotropin secretion (5,6).	2b

REFERENCES

1. Macklon NS, Stouffer RL, Giudice LC, Fauser BCJM. The science behind 25 years of ovarian stimulation for in vitro fertilization Endocrine Reviews. 2006; 27(2):170–207. doi: 10.1210/er.2005-0015.
2. Beckers NGM, Macklon NS, Fauser BCJM. Follicular and luteal phase aspects of ovarian stimulation for in vitro fertilisation. 2006; 11–3.
3. Ledger LW. Ovarian and Menstrual Cycles, Chapter 49, pp. 509–513.
4. Macklon NS, Greer IA, Steegers EAP. Textbook of Periconceptional Medicine. Chapter 21, The Luteal Phase, pp. 298–9.
5. Young J, George JT, Tello JA, Francou B, Bouligand J, Guiochon-Mantel A et al. Kisspeptin restores pulsatile LH secretion in patients with neurokinin B signaling deficiencies: Physiological, pathophysiological and therapeutic implications. Neuroendocrinology. 2013 Mar; 97(2):193–202. Published online Feb 24, 2012. doi: 10.1159/000336376 PMCID: PMC3902960.
6. Pinilla L, Aguilar E, Dieguez C, Millar RP, Tena-Sempere M. Kisspeptins and reproduction: Physiological roles and regulatory mechanisms. Physiological Reviews. 2012, July; 92(3):1235–316. doi: 10.1152/physrev.00037.2010.

2

Classification of Anovulation

Evert J. P. van Santbrink

Introduction

Oligo and anovulation represent a major cause of subfertility (LOE 3). It may either be clinically presented by a total absence of follicular development, resulting in amenorrhea, or in a disturbed development of a dominant follicle reflected by oligomenorrhea.

We consider the duration of the menstrual cycle to be normal if it is between 25 and 35 days with a median of 28 days (1). When the average duration of the menstrual cycle exceeds the 35-day limit, it is called oligomenorrhea; this is based on decreasing chances for ovulation and pregnancy when the duration of the menstrual cycle is prolonged (LOE 3; 2). We speak of amenorrhea when there is no menstrual cycle for a period of at least 6 months.

Classification

Classification of oligo or anovulation may be done in several ways: by the clinical appearance (primary or secondary), the organ of origin that causes the problem (hypothalamic, pituitary, or ovary), or the regulating system that causes the disturbance (hormonal, genetic, metabolic).

Most frequently, chronic anovulation is classified by World Health Organization (WHO) criteria, originally determined by Insler et al. (3,4). The criteria used are mean menstrual cycle duration (>35 days) and serum concentrations of follicle-stimulating hormone (FSH) and estradiol (E_2). This classification can only be used after external influences on the hypothalamic–pituitary–ovarian system are excluded, such as hyperprolactinemia, adrenal hyperandrogenism, and thyroid dysfunction (LOE 4). For practical reasons, the etiology and treatment of primary amenorrhea are outside the scope of this book.

When the origin of menstrual cycle disturbance is situated in the hypothalamus or pituitary, resulting in both decreased serum FSH and estradiol concentrations, it is classified as WHO class 1 anovulation. Another etiology of anovulation may be ovarian failure: The ovaries are functioning insufficiently, and serum FSH is elevated whereas estradiol is low. This status, also known as premature ovarian insufficiency when occurrence is before the age of 40 years, can be classified as WHO3 anovulation. The largest part (about 80%) of anovulation patients exhibit normal FSH and estradiol serum concentrations and are classified as WHO class 2. Polycystic ovary syndrome (PCOS) encompasses a subgroup of these WHO2 patients (5). The criteria for establishing the diagnosis of PCOS have been under debate for an extensive period. Criteria set by the National Institute of Health in 1992 (6) combined androgen excess and ovarian dysfunction, while polycystic morphology of the ovaries was not included. Later on, the Rotterdam consensus meeting formulated strict PCOS criteria to facilitate comparison of clinical research from different institutes around the world and improve understanding of the etiology and treatment options (7,8). These criteria were also recently acknowledged by the Endocrine Society consensus meeting (9).

Relevant criteria used for the definition of PCOS should not only be able to create a strictly defined group of patients (diagnosis based on a dysfunction of a specific organ system), but may also have predictive value on the treatment possibilities and treatment outcome (prognosis, severity of the illness). As we are increasingly aware that initial patient characteristics rather than the chosen treatment modality determine treatment success or failure, this clinical tool may enable us to apply an individually tailored treatment approach.

The Rotterdam criteria for PCOS diagnosis encompass the presence of two of the following criteria: androgen excess (biochemical or clinical), ovulatory dysfunction, or polycystic ovaries on ultrasound. Establishing the diagnosis may be complicated in adolescents and menopausal women (LOE 4). Although hyperandrogenism has a central role to the presentation in adolescents, the phenotype in postmenopausal women is less consistent. It may be concluded that using the Rotterdam criteria instead of the NIH criteria for PCOS, patients with less severe metabolic derangement will be added to the PCOS group (10).

Conclusion

The most common classification system of chronic oligo or anovulation is proposed by the WHO and based on hormonal serum concentrations of FSH and estradiol (Table 2.3). Before using this, hyperprolactinemia, adrenal hyperandrogenism and thyroid dysfunction have to be excluded. The majority of patients are classified as WHO class 2 anovulation, and a substantial number of these patients fulfill PCOS criteria. The most widely accepted criteria for PCOS diagnosis are the Rotterdam criteria.

TABLE 2.3

Endocrine Classification of Oligo and Anovulation (WHO)

WHO Classification	Hormonal Profile	Organ Involved
Class 1	Hypogonadotropic, hypo-estrogenic	Hypothalamic–pituitary
Class 2	Normogonadotropic, normo-estrogenic	Dysbalance pituitary–ovary
Class 3	Hypergonadotropic, hypo-estrogenic	Ovary

TABLE 2.1

Level of Evidence of Statements

Statement	Level of Evidence
Chronic anovulation is a major cause of subfertility.	3
Chances for ovulation and pregnancy decrease when the duration of the menstrual cycle is prolonged.	3
Establishing the diagnosis of PCOS is complicated in adolescents and menopausal women.	4
Patients with less severe metabolic derangement will be added to the PCOS group using the Rotterdam criteria instead of the NIH criteria.	3

TABLE 2.2

Grade of Strength for Recommendations

Recommendation	Grade Strength
WHO criteria should be used for classification of anovulation.	GCP
Diagnosing PCOS should be performed by using the Rotterdam criteria.	GCP

REFERENCES

1. van Santbrink EJ, Hop WC, van Dessel HJ, de Jong FH, Fauser BC. Decremental FSH and dominant follicle development during the normal menstrual cycle. Fertil Steril 1995; 64:37–43.
2. Wise LA, Mikkelsen EM, Rothman KJ, Riis AH, Sørensen HT, Huybrechts KF, Hatch EE. A prospective cohort study of menstrual characteristics and time to pregnancy. Am J Epidemiol 2011; 174(6):701–9.
3. Insler V, Melmed H, Mashiah S, Monselise M, Lunenfeld B, Rabau E. Functional classification of patients selected for gonadotropic therapy. Obstet Gynecol 1968; 32:620–6.
4. Rowe PJ, Comhaire FA, Hargreave TB, Mellow HJ. WHO manual for the standardized investigation and diagnosis of the infertile couple. Cambridge University Press, Cambridge, England. 1997; 1–80.
5. Van Santbrink EJ, Hop WC, Fauser BC. Classification of normogonadotropic infertility: Polycystic ovaries diagnosed by ultrasound versus endocrine characteristics of polycystic ovary syndrome. Fertil Steril 1997; 67:452–8.
6. Zawadzki JK, Dunaif A. Diagnostic criteria for polycystic ovary syndrome: Towards a rationale approach. In: Dunaif A, Givens JR, Haseltine FP, Merriam GR. Polycystic ovary syndrome. Blackwell Scientific Publications, Boston. 1992; 377–84.
7. PCOS consensus. The Rotterdam ESHRE/ASRM-Sponsored PCOS consensus workshop group. Revised 2003 consensus on diagnostic criteria and long-term health risks related to polycystic ovary syndrome (PCOS). Hum Reprod 2004; 19:41–7.
8. PCOS consensus. The Rotterdam ESHRE/ASRM-Sponsored PCOS consensus workshop group. Revised 2003 consensus on diagnostic criteria and long-term health risks related to polycystic ovary syndrome (PCOS). Fertil Steril 2004; 81:19–25.
9. Legro RS, Arslanian SA, Ehrmann DA, Hoeger KM, Murad MH, Pasquali R et al. Diagnosis and treatment of polycystic ovary syndrome: An Endocrine Society clinical practice guideline. J Clin Endocrinol Metab 2013 Dec; 98(12):4565–92.
10. Broekmans FJ, Knauff EA, Valkenburg O et al. PCOS according to the Rotterdam consensus criteria: Change in prevalence among WHO-II anovulation and association with metabolic factors. BJOG 2006; 1210–7.

3

Causes of Anovulation: WHO Class 1

Camille Grysole and Didier Dewailly

Introduction

WHO class 1 anovulation harbors the different anovulatory patients with a central origin (hypothalamic/pituitary) of their ovulatory dysfunction. After having easily eliminated hyperprolactinemia (HPRL) and before discussing a congenital hypogonadotropic hypogonadism (CHH), it is essential to keep in mind the other etiologies that can be either functional or organic.

According to the WHO classification, class 1 anovulation is characterized by low levels of serum estradiol and gonadotropins. However, there is an important clinical variability, and the hormonal picture is not always typical, making this diagnosis not always as easy as it seems.

Overview of Existing Evidence

The WHO class 1 anovulation results from gonadotropic insufficiency. The hormonal features of WHO class 1 anovulation include low serum estradiol levels (i.e., <30 pg/ml with the most commonly used assays) associated with low or normal serum LH and FSH levels (i.e., <2 and <4 IU/L with the most commonly used assays, respectively). Congenital and acquired causes can be distinguished (LOE 4):

→ Congenital HH (CHH):
- Kallmann syndrome
- Normosmic CHH

→ Acquired HH:
- HPRL
- Functional hypothalamic amenorrhea (FHA)
- Other causes:
  Sheehan syndrome
  Haemochromatosis
  History of cerebral radiotherapy
  Sarcoidosis
  Lymphocytic hypophysitis
  Head trauma
  Subarachnoid hemorrhage
  Cushing syndrome
  Acromegaly
  Iatrogenic HH (opiates, corticosteroids)

CHH

The prevalence of CHH, estimated between 1/10,000 and 1/14,000 in men, is considered to be two to five times lower in women. However, this frequency is underestimated due to the non-recognition of forms with partial pubertal development (LOE 4). CHH is characterized by partial or total absence of pubertal development due to inadequate secretion of pituitary gonadotropins (LH and FSH) from genetic origin in the absence of anatomic abnormalities of the hypothalamic–pituitary region and with a normal reserve of remaining pituitary hormones (1). The literature reports an increasing number of genes whose mutations are responsible for CHH. Based on the presence or absence of olfactory dysfunction, CHH is divided into two groups: CHH with olfactory impairment (called Kallmann syndrome, corresponding to abnormal migration of Gn-RH neurons with aplasia or hypoplasia of the olfactory bulbs), whose leading mutated genes are KAL1 and KAL2, and idiopathic CHH with normal olfaction (normosmic), whose most frequent mutations are in the Gn-RH-Receptor gene (1).

The diagnosis of CHH is made during the second decade of life when patients present with delayed puberty, primary or secondary amenorrhea, or during the third decade of life because of infertility. In more than 90% of cases, CHH is revealed by primary amenorrhea. The development of thelarche and adrenarche varies. It is usually present but only partially. In Kallmann syndrome, besides anosmia/hyposmia, patients can show craniofacial anomalies (cleft lip and palate, arched palate, dental agenesis, hypertelorism), neurosensorial deafness, neurological disorders (cerebellar ataxia, oculomotor disturbances, synkinesia), and digital anomalies (clinodactyly, syndactyly, camptodactyly) (1).

In CHH, it is important to exclude a HPRL by a serum prolactin measurement. It is also mandatory to evaluate all pituitary functions to eliminate an anterior hypopituitarism. Serum assays of thyroid stimulating hormone (TSH) and tetraiodothyronine (T4) allow exploring of the thyroid function. Serum insulin-like growth factor-1 (IGF-1) assesses the somatotropic axis, and morning serum cortisol and adrenocorticotropic hormone (ACTH) assays evaluate the corticotroph axis (LOE 4). Any unexplained anterior hypopituitarism requires a hypothalamic–pituitary MRI in order to detect a tumor of the hypothalamic–pituitary region. MRI with specific sections of the olfactory tract is useful in the diagnosis of Kallmann syndrome because the presence of hypoplasia or agenesis (unilateral or bilateral) of olfactory bulbs and hypoplasia of the anterior pituitary is pathognomonic of this syndrome. The genetic study must be the last step in the investigation of CHH: In the presence of hyposmia/anosmia, mutations in FGFR1, FGF8, PROK2, and PROKR2 genes must be searched first, and in case of normosmic CHH, the mutations in GN-RH1/Gn-RH receptor, KISS1R (GPR54), and TAC3/TACR3 genes are to be assessed (1). However, so far, mutations are found in only 30% of cases.

Acquired HH

HPRL

In HPRL, the partial gonadotropic insufficiency results from impaired secretion of gonadotropin-releasing hormone (Gn-RH), making it a WHO class 1 anovulation. HPRL is addressed in Chapter 7.

FHA

FHA represents 15% of the causes of secondary amenorrhea. It is the second leading cause of gonadotropic insufficiency after HPRL (LOE 4). FHA is a reversible form of Gn-RH deficiency due to a negative energy balance, which may result from dietary restriction and/or excessive physical activity (2). It is characterized by the suppression of Gn-RH pulsatility, resulting in a decreased secretion of pituitary gonadotropins, causing anovulation. Disturbances of the hypothalamic gonadal axis are associated with low leptin levels, an adipose tissue protein whose levels are proportional to fat mass and depend on calorie intake. A randomized study demonstrated that administration of recombinant human leptin allowed a recovery of menstrual cycles in these patients (LOE 2a) (3). Ghrelin, a peptide secreted by the stomach but also by the pituitary and hypothalamus, has a role in FHA: Indeed, high ghrelin levels were found in patients with FHA. Other neuropeptides are likely involved as well.

In FHA, amenorrhea usually more than 6 months, primary (for teenagers) or secondary, and is resistant to the progesterone withdrawal test. The clinical picture usually coincides with extreme weight loss, eating disorders, intensive physical practice, and psychosocial stress. Other signs can be found evoking hypo-estrogenism (vaginal dryness, libido disorders), hypometabolism (cyanosis of extremities, nervousness, lanugo hair, bradycardia, hypotension), and chronic vomiting (loss of tooth enamel, gingival abrasions, parotid gland enlargement). However, FHA is a diagnosis of exclusion (LOE 4). It is therefore necessary to look for symptoms of other causes of amenorrhea: galactorrhea, headache, visual disturbances (suggesting a central organic cause), hyperandrogenism (suggesting polycystic ovary syndrome, PCOS), premature ovarian insufficiency (POI), virilization signs such as male pattern baldness, or a clitoromegaly (suggesting adrenal hyperplasia or androgen-secreting tumor).

In FHA, the hypo-insulinemia causes an increase of sex hormone binding globulin (SHBG) and a decrease of triiodothyronine (T3), which are signs of peripheral hypometabolism (LOE 4). A minimal workup is necessary to rule out any organic cause of anovulation, such as PCOS (abnormally high serum androgens and anti-Müllerian hormone (AMH) levels, polycystic ovaries at ultrasound), POI (low AMH and estrogens, high FSH), 21-hydroxylase deficiency (abnormal high 17-hydroxyprogesterone), HPRL (abnormal high prolactin), and pituitary tumor (abnormal hypothalamic/pituitary MRI) (LOE 4).

Other Causes of Acquired HH

HH may be secondary to Sheehan syndrome, a postpartum complication related to ischemic necrosis of the anterior pituitary occurring during a postpartum hemorrhage. This syndrome has become rare with the progress of obstetrics, but it can occur in a partial form, is difficult to diagnose, and is revealed only by postpartum amenorrhea. The prevalence of pituitary deficits after brain irradiation is of the order of 80% and may occur up to 10 years after irradiation. Hypogonadism is one of the two most frequent endocrine complications of hemochromatosis with diabetes. According to the available studies in the literature, the frequency of hypogonadism is 40%–50%. Despite treatment with bloodlettings, normalization of pituitary function is exceptional. The infiltrative and inflammatory diseases of the pituitary gland can result in a gonadotropin deficit, frequently associated with other pituitary deficits. Sarcoidosis affects the central nervous system in 10% of cases, including the hypothalamic–pituitary axis in one-third of cases. Lymphocytic hypophysitis, with a prevalence of 1.9 million, mainly occurs during pregnancy or postpartum. A gonadotropic deficiency after a head injury or subarachnoid hemorrhage is present in 10%–30% of cases with no correlation to the severity of the trauma. HH may also occur in Cushing syndrome and acromegaly but can also be iatrogenic, caused by opiates or high-dose and long-term corticosteroids.

Discussion

There are diagnostic difficulties regarding WHO class 1 anovulation.

Although widely used, the diagnostic value of the Gn-RH test in CHH has been questioned because of its poor profitability. The Gn-RH test is classically positive (with preserved response of gonadotropins) in FHA, although it would be negative in CHH. Actually, it provides no additional information compared to baseline FSH and LH levels (LOE 4). Its response is variable and depends on the severity of the gonadotropin deficiency, which can be better assessed by clinical features (such as the degree of breast development), the baseline LH and FSH assays using ultrasensitive techniques, and pelvic ultrasound that allows measuring the uterus height, which is <45 mm in case of severe and long-lasting gonadotropin deficiency (LOE 4).

A hypothalamic/pituitary MRI must be performed systematically in FHA to eliminate an organic cause (essentially a pituitary or supra-pituitary tumor) (LOE 4). The existence of persistent or severe headache, non-induced vomiting, or visual disorders are late symptoms.

CHH is often underdiagnosed in patients with partial forms of the disease and who have normal breast and hair development and only chronic oligomenorrhea. Differentiating a partial form of normosmic CHH without identified mutation from FHA is sometimes challenging. Indeed, caloric restriction, related to an eating disorder, is not always revealed by the nutrition survey. A psychiatric evaluation can be helpful. In addition, both states may coexist, which could explain why all women do not have the same sensitivity to energy deficit. Indeed, some genetic mutations involved in CHH are also found in a simple heterozygous state in patients with FHA (LOE 4) (4). This is an additional difficulty in differentiating FHA from CHH.

In 30%–50% of FHA patients, a polycystic ovarian morphology can be found without real PCOS (LOE 4) (5). This can lead to erroneously diagnose PCOS and to underdiagnose FHA. In this situation, careful analysis of energy balance and serum LH assay (low to normal in FHA, normal to high in PCOS) can help.

Conclusion

WHO class 1 anovulation is a common cause of infertility, and each cause should be assessed because it requires specific treatments. For ovulation induction, the specific treatment is pulsatile administration of Gn-RH that is relatively easy, providing appropriate devices are used (see Chapter 14).

However, these diseases are often underdiagnosed. Indeed, the clinical presentation as well as the hormonal picture shows considerable variation. This variability must be known not to underestimate their diagnosis.

Nevertheless, research to improve their identification is constantly evolving, especially in the field of genetics.

TABLE 3.1

Level of Evidence of Statements

Statement	Level of Evidence
WHO class 1 anovulation results from either congenital or acquired causes.	4
Based on the presence or absence of an olfaction defect, CHH is divided into two groups: CHH with anosmia/hyposmia and idiopathic CHH with normal olfaction.	4
Beside anosmia/hyposmia, Kallmann syndrome may include craniofacial, neurosensorial, and dysmorphic anomalies.	4
FHA represents 15% of cases of secondary amenorrhea and is the second leading cause of acquired HH after hyperprolactinemia.	4
FHA is a reversible form of GnRH deficiency due to a negative energy balance.	4
30%–50% of patients with FHA have polycystic ovarian morphology at ultrasound without real PCOS.	4

TABLE 3.2

Grade of Strength for Recommendations

Recommendation	Grade Strength
In CHH, it is important to evaluate all pituitary functions to eliminate an anterior hypopituitarism.	D
The genetic study is often the last step in the investigation of the CHH.	D
Although widely used, the diagnostic value of the GnRH test in CHH has been questioned because of its low profitability.	D
Hypothalamic/pituitary MRI must be performed systematically in FHA.	GPP
A psychiatric evaluation can be helpful for diagnosing an eating disorder.	GPP
The baseline serum LH assay can help differentiate FHA from PCOS.	GPP

REFERENCES

1. Silveira LF, Latronico AC. Approach of the patient with hypogonadotropic hypogonadism. J Clin Endocrinol Metab. 2013; 98(5):1781–8.
2. Catherine M, Gordon MD. 2010. Clinical practice. Functional Hypothalamic Amenorrhea. N Engl J Med. 2010, July; (363):365–71.
3. Welt CK, Chan JL, Bullen J. Recombinant human leptin in women with hypothalamic amenorrhea. N Engl J Med. 2004; (351):987–97.
4. Caronia LM, Martin C, Welt CK. 2011. A genetic basis for functional hypothalamic amenorrhea. N Engl J Med. 2011; (364):215–25.
5. Robin G, Gallo C, Catteau-Jonard S, Lefebvre-Maunoury C, Pigny P, Duhamel A, Dewailly D. Polycystic ovary-like abnormalities (PCO-L) in women with functional hypothalamic amenorrhea. J Clin Endocrinol Metab. 2012; 97(11):4236–43.

4

Causes of Anovulation: Normogonadotropic Normoestrogenic Anovulation Non-PCOS

Sharon V. Lie Fong and Yvonne V. Louwers

Introduction

The majority of anovulatory women present with normal serum gonadotrophin levels and normal estradiol levels. Of these women, about 10% do not comply with diagnostic criteria for polycystic ovary syndrome (PCOS) according to the Rotterdam consensus (1). Whether or not this should be recognized as a subgroup with a different etiology and prognosis will be discussed further on.

Overview of Existing Evidence

Normogonadotropic anovulation is the most frequent cause of anovulatory infertility and includes women with a heterogeneous phenotype. Because the vast majority of normogonadotropic women has PCOS, WHO 2 anovulation non-PCOS can only be diagnosed after Rotterdam PCOS characteristics have been ruled out (1). This may be challenging in women with hirsutism or acne but normal serum androgen levels, such as in the following conditions:

- Idiopathic hirsutism: This is a rather common disorder. Serum androgens are normal, and there is no other identifiable cause for the hirsutism.
- Drug use: Oligomenorrhea and hirsutism are known side effects of corticosteroids and valproic acid. Progestins, such as danazol, can cause acne. Minoxidil is an antihypertensive drug that may cause hirsutism. This has also been described in the use of the anti-epileptic drug phenytoin and phenothiazine, a tricyclic antidepressant.

The diagnosis of less common disorders that may cause signs of virilization due to increased serum androgen levels may be even more difficult. These disorders include the following:

- Late-onset congenital adrenal hyperplasia (see Chapter 7)
- Androgen-secreting tumors in the ovary
  - Sertoli-Leydig cell tumor: This type of ovarian tumor accounts for less than 0.5% of all ovarian tumors. It has a low grade of malignancy and presents unilaterally. It can occur at all ages but usually during the second and third decade. In 70%–80% of women with this type of tumor, increased testosterone levels may cause progressive virilization.
- Tumors in the adrenal gland
  - Adenoma of the adrenal cortex are common tumors of the adrenal gland. Only 15% of these tumors are functional. Excessive cortisol production typically causes Cushing's

syndrome. Occasionally, androgen production also increases, and in these patients, hirsutism and acne may be present.

- Adrenocortical carcinoma is extremely rare. The incidence is estimated 0.5–2 per million per year, and about 50% of the tumors produce steroids.

- Ovarian hyperthecosis: This condition usually affects postmenopausal women. It is characterized by the presence of bilateral enlarged ovaries due to stromal hyperplasia and luteinization of theca cells. The hyperplastic cells produce excessive androgens, resulting in increased serum androgen levels and progressive signs of hirsutism and virilization. Most women report regular menstrual cycles in the past and have never been diagnosed with PCOS (2).

Finally, other endocrine causes of anovulation should be excluded:

- Thyroid disorders (see Chapter 8).
- Hyperprolactinemia (see Chapter 9).
- Chronic renal disease: Anovulatory infertility may occur due to increased ureum levels in women with end stage renal disease.
- Insulin resistance: A rare condition of severe tissue resistance to insulin, associated with hyperandrogenism and acanthosis nigricans. These symptoms have been described in young women with type A syndrome caused by mutations in the insulin signaling system. Women with type B syndrome are older women with immunologic disease. Insulin resistance in these women is caused by auto-antibodies to the insulin receptor.

Discussion

Exclusion of PCOS is of great importance because of the possible long-term consequences of the syndrome (3). It seems plausible that some long-term consequences for general health described in women with PCOS, for example, development of endometrial pathology due to unopposed estrogen exposure, may also apply to WHO 2 non-PCOS women. So far, the long-term health consequences have not been studied in normogonadotropic women without PCOS (4).

In order to correctly diagnose normogonadotropic normoestrogenic anovulation without PCOS in women presenting with oligomenorrhea, hirsutism, and virilization, careful history-taking on the onset and progression of symptoms, medical history, and drug use is essential. With aging and consequently with decrease of the ovarian reserve, anovulatory women may regain regular menstrual cycles (5). If transvaginal ultrasound imaging and initial endocrine screening are insufficient, an ACTH stimulation test and dexamethasone suppression test may provide additional information in the differentiation of the ovarian or adrenal source of hyperandrogenism.

Treatment of cycle irregularity in non-PCOS anovulation includes oral contraceptives or induction of withdrawal bleedings on a regular basis. In hyperandrogenic non-PCOS women, hirsutism may ameliorate with oral contraceptives containing cyproterone acetate. Other anti-androgenic drugs, such as spironolactone or finasteride, are also effective but are teratogenic and therefore less suitable for women of reproductive age. When medication alone does not decrease excessive hair growth sufficiently, combination with hair removal techniques may be required.

Conclusions

Normogonadotropic normoestrogenic anovulation non-PCOS is only diagnosed after exclusion of PCOS and other endocrinological causes of anovulation.

TABLE 4.1

Level of Evidence of Statements

Statement	Level of Evidence
Most anovulatory women with normal gonadotrophin and estradiol levels have PCOS.	3
Normogonadotropic normoestrogenic anovulation without PCOS may be caused by other endocrine disorders, for example, thyroid disease, hyperprolactinemia, pathology of the adrenal gland.	3
Long-term health consequences in women with normogonadotropic normoestrogenic anovulation but without PCOS are unknown.	4

TABLE 4.2

Grade of Strength for Recommendations

Recommendation	Grade Strength
In normogonadotropic anovulatory women, the presence of PCOS should be excluded.	GPP
After exclusion of PCOS, the presence of endocrinological disorders should be excluded by history-taking, pelvic ultrasound, and endocrine screening.	GPP

REFERENCES

1. Broekmans FJ, Knauff EA, Valkenburg O, Laven JS, Eijkemans MJ, Fauser BC. PCOS according to the Rotterdam consensus criteria: Change in prevalence among WHO-II anovulation and association with metabolic factors. Bjog. 2006; 113:1210–7.
2. Alpanes M, Gonzalez-Casbas JM, Sanchez J, Pian H, Escobar-Morreale HF. Management of postmenopausal virilization. Journal Clin Endocrinol Metab. 2012; 97:2584–8.
3. Fauser BC, Tarlatzis BC, Rebar RW, Legro RS, Balen AH, Lobo R et al. Consensus on women's health aspects of polycystic ovary syndrome (PCOS): The Amsterdam ESHRE/ASRM-Sponsored 3rd PCOS Consensus Workshop Group. Fertil Steril. 2012; 97:28–38, e25.
4. ESHRE Capri Workshop Group. Health and fertility in World Health Organization group 2 anovulatory women. Hum Reprod Update. 2012; 18:586–99.
5. Brown ZA, Louwers YV, Lie Fong S, Valkenburg O, Birnie E, de Jong FH et al. The phenotype of polycystic ovary syndrome ameliorates with aging. Fertil Steril. 2011; 96:1259–65.

5

Causes of Anovulation: WHO Type 2: Polycystic Ovary Syndrome

Richard S. Legro

Introduction

WHO Type 2 ovulatory dysfunction is characterized by disordered hypothalmic–pituitary–ovarian communication and function. PCOS classically presents with oligomenorrhea and signs of androgen excess, usually hirsutism. It represents the most common cause of ovulatory dysfunction, and it is estimated that 80% of cases of oligomenorrhea and oligo-ovulation are due to polycystic ovary syndrome. It is difficult to ascertain whether the prevalence of PCOS is increasing in both developed and developing countries with increasing rates of obesity or whether increased recognition of the syndrome (or looser diagnostic criteria) are leading to an "epidemic" of polycystic ovary syndrome. The cause of PCOS is unknown. The evidence for intrauterine effects on development of PCOS is inconclusive and genetic studies, including GWAS, have identified several significant associations with several genetic variants, which unfortunately only account for a small proportion of the phenotype. In this chapter, we review diagnostic criteria and associated morbidities, including suggested evaluation of women with PCOS.

Overview of Existing Evidence for the Diagnosis and Evaluation of Women with PCOS

There are a variety of diagnostic criteria for PCOS, and many societies have made recommendations (1). All of these are expert based. But all agree that PCOS remains a diagnosis of exclusion. The most popular are the Rotterdam criteria (2), which recommends that the diagnosis of PCOS be made if two of the three following criteria are met: androgen excess (either biochemical based on elevated circulating testosterone levels or clinical based in hirustism), ovulatory dysfunction (usually based on patient's self-report of menstrual history), or polycystic ovaries (usually diagnosed by transvaginal ultrasound of the basis of an elevated antral follicle count, usually >12 or an increased ovarian volume, usually >10 cm³). Because only two of three criteria need to be present, it is possible to make a diagnosis without a transvaginal ultrasound exam or, for that matter, without a serum testosterone level. At the same time, disorders that mimic the clinical features of PCOS should be excluded. These include in all women thyroid disease, hyperprolactinemia, and nonclassic congenital adrenal hyperplasia (primarily 21-hydroxylase deficiency by serum 17-OHP). In select women with amenorrhea and more severe phenotypes, for example, evidence of virilization, more extensive evaluation to identify other causes is indicated.

There are significant differences in phenotype according to race and ethnicity. For example, East Asian women may be unlikely to develop signs of clinical androgen excess, such as hirsutism and acne, despite having similar elevations in circulating testosterone levels as Caucasian women with PCOS (who present with hirsutism). Women of color may be more prone to metabolic abnormalities even if normal weight. Obesity in women with PCOS is also more prevalent among wealthy countries, most commonly the United States. Obesity can worsen both reproductive and metabolic aspects of PCOS.

The diagnosis of PCOS in adolescents is even more problematic. The diagnosis should be based on the presence of clinical and/or biochemical evidence of hyperandrogenism in the presence of persistent oligomenorrhea (oligomenorrhea can be a normal transition for 1–2 years post menarche). Hyperandrogenemia remains difficult to diagnose in adolescents because there are no age or Tanner stage specific cutoffs. Many testosterone assays have poor accuracy as levels approach normal female levels. Experts have recommended using mass spectrometry to measure testosterone levels in women because of the increased accuracy, but even these assays suffer from the same imprecision at low levels. Polycystic ovaries remains a nonspecific criterion for adolescents and young women as 20%–40% may meet criteria for polycystic ovaries given the large number of antral follicles common after menarche (3).

Recently, there has been discussion whether circulating anti-Mullerian hormone (AMH), which correlates directly with the number of antral follicles, could be used to diagnose polycystic ovaries in lieu of an ultrasound exam (4). Much of the debate about the diagnosis centers around which criteria identify the most metabolically challenged women, and generally, phenotypes that focus on the clinical criteria of androgen excess and oligomenorrhea tend to have higher prevalence of metabolic syndrome and glucose intolerance. There are currently no diagnostic criteria for PCOS in peri- and menopausal women. Part of the difficulty in diagnosing PCOS in older women is the fact that the ovary fails eventually in all women, so that androgen levels, ovarian volume, and antral follicle count decrease with age. There are data, however, to suggest that the larger initial cohort of follicles in women with PCOS may mean a slightly later menopause (5).

Evaluation and Counseling of Women with PCOS

Physical examination should search for cutaneous manifestations of PCOS: terminal hair growth acne, alopecia, acanthosis nigricans (often associated with hyperinsulinemia), and skin tags. Increased adiposity, particularly abdominal, is associated with hyperandrogenemia and increased metabolic risk; therefore, BMI and waist measurements should be obtained. Signs of hypercortisolism, including moon facies, buffalo hump, abdominal striae, and proximal muscle weakness (difficulty in rising from a chair) should trigger concern for possible Cushing's syndrome. Given the low prevalence of this syndrome and the chance for false positive findings on screening tests, routine screening for Cushing's is not indicated in women with PCOS.

Women with PCOS are at increased risk of anovulation and infertility; in the absence of anovulation, for example, in the woman with PCOS based on polycystic ovaries and hyperandrogenism, the risk of infertility is uncertain. Although anovulatory infertility is assumed to be the primary cause of infertility, other causes may be present in the couple, and therefore routine evaluation of the male factor and tubal factor is indicated. One large randomized controlled study showed that 10% of couples presenting with presumed anovulatory infertility due to PCOS also had significant oligospermia (6). Infertility may be more common among younger women with PCOS; long-term follow-up studies suggest that most women with PCOS conceive, and their number of children is similar to other women. Because women with PCOS are at increased risk of pregnancy complications (gestational diabetes, preterm delivery, and preeclampsia) exacerbated by obesity, women should be counseled and also assessed preconception for BMI, blood pressure, and oral glucose tolerance (7).

Menstrual abnormalities range from amenorrhea to abnormal uterine bleeding and are a frequent presenting complaint. Although, most times, this is due to anovulatory bleeding, endometrial pathology, including uterine polyps and endometrial hyperplasia, must also be considered. Obesity, hyperinsulinism, diabetes, and dysfunctional uterine bleeding are associated both with PCOS and increased risk of endometrial cancer. Although the data linking increased event rates of women with PCOS to endometrial cancer are stronger than that for increased cardiovascular events, similar concerns about the lack of long-term follow-up of large cohorts is present. There is, however, no recommended screening test for endometrial cancer as both transvaginal ultrasound and routine endometrial biopsy have poor sensitivity and specificity for diagnosing endometrial cancer. Although it is unlikely that obesity, per se, can cause PCOS, obesity is associated with decreases in sex hormone binding globulin, which could increase bioavailable androgen levels throughout the body (8).

Although women with PCOS clearly have increased risk factors for cardiovascular disease, the data do not support an earlier onset or a lifetime higher prevalence of cardiovascular events (9). The reasons for this discrepancy are uncertain, but lack of long-term longitudinal data hampers our ability to draw conclusions. Nonetheless, women with PCOS should receive cardiovascular risk stratification by screening for the following cardiovascular disease risk factors, which appear to be more common among women with PCOS: family history of early cardiovascular disease, cigarette smoking, impaired glucose tolerance or type 2 diabetes mellitus, hypertension, dyslipidemia, obstructive sleep apnea, and obesity (10). Women with PCOS are at increased risk for glucose intolerance and diabetes even if normal weight. They should be screened with preferably a 75-g oral glucose tolerance test, but if unable, a glycohemoglobin level should be obtained. Women should likely be rescreened over time, but the optimal interval has not been established although experts have recommended every 3–5 years. It is important to note that most women with PCOS, even those with impaired glucose tolerance, will have normal fasting glucose levels, and this test alone is likely insensitive for screening for eventual diabetes risk (11). Similarly, insulin levels have little clinical significance, and routine screening of insulin levels is not recommended.

Smoking appears to be more common among women with PCOS than other women. Smoking has been associated with altered testosterone levels and exacerbations of insulin sensitivity. There are a variety of other metabolic disorders as noted above, likely related to insulin resistance that may affect women with PCOS. Dyslipidemia may be the most common metabolic abnormality, and up to 50% of women will display at least one abnormal lipid level by U.S. National Cholesterol Education Program (NCEP) guidelines. Most commonly, these are LDL elevations and triglyceride elevations. Thus, all women should be screened with a fasting lipid profile. Sleep abnormalities, including disordered sleep breathing and sleep apnea, are also more common. When symptoms (for example, daytime sleepiness or snoring) exist, patients should be screened with polysomnography, but routine polysomnography is likely not indicated. Women may also be more prone to developing nonalcoholic fatty liver disease (NAFLD) and nonalcoholic steatohepatitis (NASH). Routine screening of liver function is not indicated given the uncertainty of the long-term prognosis. Finally, women with PCOS have an increased incidence of mood disorders, including anxiety and depression, and symptoms should be routinely queried on initial exam. Many of the signs and symptoms of PCOS, for example, infertility, obesity, and male pattern hair distribution, are highly correlated with decreased quality of life and likely contribute to mood disorders (12).

Conclusion

PCOS is the most common cause of ovulatory dysfunction and is a leading cause of human infertility. Although the diagnosis can usually be made by history and physical exam, ultrasound exam and hormonal assays can assist in the diagnosis. Women with PCOS should be evaluated for associated reproductive and metabolic dysfunction.

TABLE 5.1

Level of Evidence of Statements

Statement	Level of Evidence
PCOS is diagnosed by two of these three criteria: hyperandrogenism, oligomenorrhea, or polycystic ovaries.	5
Oligomenorrhea and polycystic ovaries are common among adolescent women and confound the diagnosis in this age group.	2
Women with PCOS are at increased risk for infertility.	1a
Women with PCOS share many of the risk factors for endometrial cancer and may be at increased risk.	3a
Obesity is associated with increased metabolic risk and hyperandrogenism.	1a
Women with PCOS have an increased prevalence of anxiety and depression.	2a
Women with PCOS have an increased prevalence of cardiovascular risk factors, including family history of early cardiovascular disease, cigarette smoking, impaired glucose tolerance or type 2 diabetes, hypertension, dyslipidemia, obstructive sleep apnea, and obesity (especially increased abdominal adiposity).	2a
Despite the adverse cardiometabolic profile, there are not clear data supporting early onset or increase prevalence of cardiovascular events.	2c

TABLE 5.2

Grade of Strength for Recommendations

Recommendation	Grade Strength
Other mimics, such as thyroid disease, prolactin excess, and congenital adrenal hyperplasia (21-hydroxylase deficiency), should be routinely excluded.	B
Rare causes of similar symptoms, such as Cushing's syndrome, androgen secreting tumor, or steroid abuse, should be selectively excluded.	B
Women with PCOS should not undergo routine screening with ultrasound or biopsy for endometrial cancer.	C
Women with PCOS should undergo routine screening for dysglycemia with an oral glucose tolerance test or a glycohemoglobin level.	A
Women with PCOS should undergo routine screening with a fasting lipid profile.	A
Women with PCOS should be selectively screened for sleep disorders and liver disease.	C
Other infertility factors should be considered in couples presenting with infertility presumed secondary to female PCOS-related anovulation.	A

REFERENCES

1. Legro RS, Arslanian SA, Ehrmann DA, Hoeger KM, Murad MH, Pasquali R et al. Diagnosis and treatment of polycystic ovary syndrome: An Endocrine Society clinical practice guideline. J Clin Endocrinol Metab. 2013 Dec; 98(12):4565–92. PubMed PMID: 24151290
2. Revised 2003 consensus on diagnostic criteria and long-term health risks related to polycystic ovary syndrome (PCOS). Hum Reprod. 2004 Jan; 19(1):41–7. PubMed PMID: 14688154
3. Johnstone EB, Rosen MP, Neril R, Trevithick D, Sternfeld B, Murphy R et al. The polycystic ovary post-Rotterdam: A common, age-dependent finding in ovulatory women without metabolic significance. J Clin Endocrinol Metab. 2010 Nov; 95(11):4965–72. PubMed PMID: 20719841. Pubmed Central PMCID: 2968725. Epub 2010/08/20. eng.
4. Pigny P, Jonard S, Robert Y, Dewailly D. Serum anti-Mullerian hormone as a surrogate for antral follicle count for definition of the polycystic ovary syndrome. J Clin Endocrinol Metab. 2006 Mar; 91(3):941–5. PubMed PMID: 16368745. Epub 2005/12/22. eng.
5. Tehrani FR, Solaymani-Dodaran M, Hedayati M, Azizi F. Is polycystic ovary syndrome an exception for reproductive aging? Hum Reprod. 2010 Jul; 25(7):1775–81. PubMed PMID: 20435693. Epub 2010/05/04. eng.

6. Legro RS, Barnhart HX, Schlaff WD, Carr BR, Diamond MP, Carson SA et al. Clomiphene, metformin, or both for infertility in the polycystic ovary syndrome. N Engl J Med. 2007 Feb; 356(6):551–66. PubMed PMID: 17287476

7. Boomsma CM, Eijkemans MJ, Hughes EG, Visser GH, Fauser BC, Macklon NS. A meta-analysis of pregnancy outcomes in women with polycystic ovary syndrome. Hum Reprod Update. 2006 Aug 4. PubMed PMID: 16891296

8. Legro RS, Dodson WC, Gnatuk CL, Estes SJ, Kunselman AR, Meadows JW et al. Effects of gastric bypass surgery on female reproductive function. J Clin Endocrinol Metabol. 2012 Dec; 97(12):4540–8. PubMed PMID: 23066115. Pubmed Central PMCID: 3513539

9. Polotsky AJ, Allshouse AA, Crawford SL, Harlow SD, Khalil N, Kazlauskaite R et al. Hyperandrogenic oligomenorrhea and metabolic risks across menopausal transition. J Clin Endocrinol Metabol. 2014 Jun; 99(6):2120–7. PubMed PMID: 24517154. Pubmed Central PMCID: 4037727

10. Diamanti-Kandarakis E, Dunaif A. Insulin resistance and the polycystic ovary syndrome revisited: An update on mechanisms and implications. Endocr Rev. 2012 Dec; 33(6):981–1030. PubMed PMID: 23065822

11. Legro RS, Kunselman AR, Dodson WC, Dunaif A. Prevalence and predictors of risk for type 2 diabetes mellitus and impaired glucose tolerance in polycystic ovary syndrome: A prospective, controlled study in 254 affected women. J Clin Endocrinol Metabol. 1999; 84(1):165–9.

12. Veltman-Verhulst SM, Boivin J, Eijkemans MJ, Fauser BJ. Emotional distress is a common risk in women with polycystic ovary syndrome: A systematic review and meta-analysis of 28 studies. Hum Reprod Update. 2012 Nov–Dec; 18(6):638–51. PubMed PMID: 22824735. Epub 2012/07/25. eng.

6

Causes of Anovulation: WHO Class 3

Sophie Christin-Maitre and Jean-Pierre Siffroi

Introduction

WHO class 3 anovulation is characterized by hypergonadotropic hypogonadism or primary ovarian insufficiency, and is also called premature ovarian insufficiency (POI). POI (MIM 311360) is diagnosed in adolescents with primary amenorrhea or in adolescents or young women presenting with secondary amenorrhea lasting more than 6 months and occurring before the age of 40. In all cases, plasma gonadotropins are in the postmenopausal range, and estradiol levels are low (1). Classically, FSH serum levels, measured twice, at least 1 month apart, are higher than 40 IU/L. ESHRE guidelines recommend an elevated FSH level >25 IU/L on two occasions >4 weeks apart (2). In most cases, the antral follicle count (AFC) evaluated by pelvic ultrasound examination is diminished, and AMH serum level is very low (LOE 2a).

Overview of Existing Evidence

POI affects 1%–3% of reproductive-age women (LOE 3). POI should be distinguished from diminished ovarian reserve (DOR). Indeed, women with DOR have infertility associated with antral follicular counts below 10, but they are still menstruating. Furthermore, their FSH levels are only slightly elevated and not in the menopausal range. The term POI is more accurate than premature ovarian failure (POF) or premature menopause. Indeed, the term menopause suggests a definitive arrest of ovarian function, and variable degrees of ovarian function are preserved in a subset of patients with POI. Second, hormonal replacement therapy (HRT) is necessary for women with POI in order to avoid effects related to estrogen deficiency. Finally, the term POI is less stigmatizing. Among the different etiologies of POI, genetic causes should be distinguished from infectious, surgical, and toxic causes.

Among the toxic causes, chemotherapy and radiotherapy are becoming frequent causes of POI due to a growing population of childhood/adolescent cancer survivors (3). Alkylating agents remain some of the most toxic drugs as they induce POI in 40%–50% of treated women. Sixty to eighty percent of women treated with cyclophosphamide, methotrexate, and 5-fluorouracil will develop POI. Chemotherapeutic agents damage the ovary by increasing follicle loss (3). This phenomenon can be due to direct damage to the oocytes and direct damage to somatic cells as well as an increased rate of follicle growth initiation (3). The impact of radiotherapy is dependent on dose, age at treatment, and on the radiation therapy field. Many occupational exposures to chemicals have been shown to induce POI in animal models (4). However, in humans, environmental causes are difficult to identify. A study has reported an adjusted RR of POI of 3.24 (1.06–9.9) in hairdressers using dyes without gloves (5).

Cases of POI have been reported after ovarian surgery or uterine artery embolization. A potential detrimental effect of surgery has been described mainly in patients operated for bilateral ovarian endometriomas (6). The laparoscopic stripping of recurrent ovarian endometriomas has been associated with a high risk of ovarian failure. Furthermore, endometriosis by itself could influence ovarian aging and increase the risk of POI (LOE 3).

In the absence of previous chemotherapy, radiotherapy, or ovarian surgery, genetic causes of POI need to be investigated (1). Some genetic causes of POI are syndromic (Table 6.3). Most of them are linked to X chromosomal abnormalities. They include abnormal numbers as well as structural defects of the X chromosomes. The most common is Turner syndrome with 45, X karyotype, 45,X/46,XX mosaicism or Xq isochromosome. Clinical features of Turner syndrome include small height and ovarian insufficiency. Around 30%–40% of patients with Turner syndrome enter puberty, but less than 10% have spontaneous menses and more than 95% will develop POI (7). Among patients with Turner syndrome, the diagnosis is established in adults in 10% of cases. In POI, apart from Turner syndrome, the karyotype can also reveal Xq deletions as well as X;autosomal translocations or trisomy X. By studying patients with Xq deletions, it has been demonstrated that two different regions located on the long arm of the X chromosome are necessary for the maintenance of ovarian follicles. Those regions, named POF1 and POF2, are able to escape X inactivation (8). Therefore, in case of haplo-insufficiency, ovarian follicle loss is accelerated. In X;autosome translocations, most breakpoints concern desert gene regions, thus suggesting underlying mechanisms different than gene mutations. A position effect on autosomes translocated on the X chromosome and, more recently, epigenetic effects on the long arm of the X chromosome have been suggested (9). Taken together, X chromosome abnormalities represent around 10%–15% of POI (LOE 2a).

POI is associated with familial or personal history of autoimmune diseases in 4%–5% of POI cases (LOE 3). It belongs to autoimmune polyendocrinopathy syndromes (APS). APS type 1 stands for autoimmune polyendocrinopathy candidosis ectodermal dystrophy syndrome (APECED). It is related to autosomal recessive *AIRE* gene mutations (10). In type 2 APS, patients present with type 1 diabetes mellitus, adrenal insufficiency, and hypothyroidism. POI is present in 10%–25% of APS-2 patients. In APS type 4, patients have vitiligo, systemic lupus erythematosus, and chronic atrophic gastritis. An Italian study has shown that in all cases of APS, Addison disease occurs at an earlier age than POI (11). Genes involved in APS-2 and APS-4 have not been identified so far. In autoimmune POI, cases of serum LH levels may be higher than FSH levels (12). Furthermore, in autoimmune POI, the numbers of ovarian follicles and AMH levels are higher than in non-autoimmune POI (13). Autoimmunity seems to induce selective theca cell destruction, preserving granulosa cell function (LOE 2a). Very few cases of POI, apart from autoimmune causes, are associated with high AMH levels. In those cases, impaired folliculogenesis is probably involved (14).

TABLE 6.3

Syndromic POI

Chromosome	Gene	Transmission	Syndrome or Associated Disease
X chrosomosome (45X; 46XX, 45X; X isochromosome)			Turner syndrome
3q23	*FOXL2*	AD	BPES
9p13	*GALT*	AR	Galactosemia
10q26	*SYCE1*	AR	Eye disease
21q22	*AIRE*	AR	APECED
5q23.1	*HSD17B4/DBP*	AR	Perrault syndrome
5q31	*HARS2*	AR	Perrault syndrome
14q24, 2p23,	*EIF2B2,4,5*	AR	White substance disease
8q21	*NBN/NBS1*	AR	Nijmegen breakage
20p12	*MCM8*	AR	Chromosomal instability
6p22	*MCM9*	AR	Chromosomal instability and short stature
11q22	*ATM*	AD	Ataxia telangectasia
			In the family
Xq27.3	*FMR1*		Fragile X syndrome
Xq28	*FMR2*		Fragile X syndrome
11q13	*NR5A1*	AD	46 XY DSD

In less than 1% of POI, patients have eyelid abnormalities and a previous history of eyelid surgery. In such cases, POI is associated with blepharophimosis–ptosis–epicanthus syndrome (BPES), an autosomal dominant syndrome. The candidate gene is *FOXL2*, encoding a protein involved in early stages of folliculogenesis (15). In 50% of BPES cases, *FOXL2* mutations are de novo (LOE 2a). In the remaining cases, they are transmitted essentially by the father as FOXL2 is not expressed in the testis and does not impair male fertility. Another ocular disease has been recently associated with an autosomal recessive form of POI. Those patients have bilateral mild nanophtalmos associated with macular dystrophy. In those cases, POI is due to *SYCE1* mutation. This gene encodes synaptonemal complex central element protein 1, a component of the synaptonemal complex involved in meiosis.

Perrault syndrome is characterized by sensorineural deafness and POI. Type I is devoid of neurological signs, and type II is associated with progressive neurological disease associating ataxia, nystagmus, ophtalmoplegia, and hypotonia. Several candidate genes have been identified in Perrault syndrome, such as *HSD17B4* and *HARS2*.

POI may be associated with white matter abnormalities at magnetic resonance imaging in relation with eukaryotic initiation factor 2B mutations (*eIF2B*). Those patients develop neurological deterioration. POI has also been associated with ataxia telangiectasia syndrome (*ATM* gene) as well as Nijmegen breakage syndrome (*NBN/NBS1 gene*). Very recently, chromosomal instability has been associated with POI. Exome sequencing in consanguineous families has revealed *MCM8* and *MCM9* mutations (16). Those genes encode minichromosomal maintenance proteins participating in DNA replication. Patients with *MCM9* mutations have short stature.

In some cases, POI is not syndromic but is associated with diseases in the family. Mental retardation in males should be searched for. Indeed, 20% of women carrying premutation of *FRAXA* or *FMR1*, the gene involved in fragile X syndrome, have POI (16) (LOE 2a). Fragile X syndrome is due to an abnormal number of CGG triplets, located at 5' of the *FMR1* gene, in Xq28. Normal individuals have less than 50 triplets, and individuals carrying a premutation have between 50 and 200 triplets. Premutated X chromosomes undergo a drastic modification when transmitted through female meiosis, leading to a full mutation characterized by more than 200 CGG triplets and by an abnormal methylation of the DNA. Full mutations are associated with the fragile X syndrome in males. Different studies have shown that *FMR1* premutations are identified in 3% of sporadic POI cases and in 13% of familial cases of POI (17). The higher risk for POI is located between 80 and 99 triplets (LOE 2a). The main mechanism involved in women with premutation is an increased *FMR1* mRNA transcription inducing oocyte as well as granulosa cell toxicity and therefore POI.

Another syndrome, potentially present in the family, is 46 XY disorder of sexual development (DSD). Indeed, *SF1* (*NR5A1*) mutations have been initially identified in four different families associating 46 XY DSD and POI (18). Since the original report, four worldwide studies have shown that the prevalence of SF1 mutations is less than 2% of sporadic cases of POI (LOE 2a).

In recent years, several non-syndromic causes of POI have been identified using linkage analysis, animal models, or more recently, whole exome sequencing in large consanguineous families (Table 6.4). Those candidate genes code for proteins involved in folliculogenesis. Among the proteins expressed in granulosa cells, rare cases of FSH receptor mutations have been reported. Among the proteins expressed in oocytes, the mutations that have been identified are *GDF9* (growth differentiation factor 9), *BMP15* (19) (bone morphogenic protein), and *NOBOX* (newborn ovary homeobox). Recent data suggest that *NOBOX* mutations are quite frequent as they have been identified in 6%–7% of sporadic cases of POI in two different cohorts (20) (LOE 2a). Variants of the AMH gene with a drastically reduced in vitro bioactivity have been identified in a small cohort of POI patients.

A whole exome sequencing study in a family, including seven cases of POI, has recently identified a heterozygous stop codon in the eukaryotic translation initiation factor 4E nuclear import factor 1 (eIF4ENIF1) (21). In this family, this autosomal dominant non-sense mutation segregated with the disease. This protein is expressed in the oocyte and plays a role in ovarian germ cell development. A potential mechanism involved could be haploinsufficiency, resulting in decreased mRNA degradation and mRNA instability. This study illustrates the importance of translation initiation factors and their regulators in ovarian function. The most recent candidate genes identified in POI are involved in meiosis. A homozygous 1-bp deletion in the gene encoding stromal antigen 3 (STAG3) was identified in a consanguineous Palestinian family, including five cases of primary amenorrhea. *STAG3* encodes a

TABLE 6.4

Non-Syndromic Causes of POI

Chromosome	Gene
Xq deletions	
X, autosome translocation	
Xp11	*BMP15*
Xq21	*DIAPH2*
Xq22	*PGRMC1*
1p22	*HFM1*
2p21	*FSHR*
2p13	*FIGLA*
5q31	*GDF9*
6q21	*FOXO3a*
7p15	*INHA*
7q22	*STAG3*
7q25	*NOBOX*
9q	*elF4ENIF1*
15q21	*CYP19A1*
15q25	*CPEB1*
16p13	*PMM2*
19p13	*NANOS3*
22q13	*DMC1*

meiosis-specific subunit of the cohesin ring, involved in sister chromatin cohesion (22). The prevalence of *STAG3* mutation in sporadic cases remains unknown. Heterozygous mutations in the *HFM1* gene have been described in two Chinese sisters. This gene encodes a protein regulating meiosis. Microdeletions of *CPEB1* gene have been recently reported (23).

During follow-up of patients with POI, clinicians should be aware of possible waxing and waning ovarian function (LOE 2a). Spontaneous pregnancies have been described in 4%–6% of patients. Hormonal replacement therapy should be advised at least until the physiological age of menopause.

In summary, POI is a very heterogeneous disorder. More than 30 genes have been identified as candidate genes in POI (Tables 6.3 and 6.4), and the list keeps expanding. Next-generation sequencing (NGS) is now simplifying the search for POI etiologies as many genes can be tested at the same time. However, the cause of POI remains unidentified in more than 70% of cases. In summary, the tests to be performed in women presenting with WHO 3 anovulation are FSH serum levels performed twice, a karyotype, a search for *FMR1* premutation, TSH, antithyroid antibodies, 21-hydroxylase antibodies, and when available, NGS. Further research based on comparative genomic hybridization (CGH) arrays, identifying gene deletion, or gene duplication as well as whole exome sequencing in sporadic or familial cases are going to improve the number of candidate genes identified in POI in the near future.

TABLE 6.1

Level of Evidence of Statements

Statement	Level of Evidence
Alkylating agents induce POI in 40%–50% of women.	3
Chemotherapeutic agents damage the ovary by increasing follicle loss.	2b
The most common genetic cause of POI is chromosome X abnormalities.	2b
POF1 and POF2 regions located on Xq chromosome are necessary for ovarian follicle maintenance.	2a
POI is associated with familial or personal history of autoimmune diseases in 4%–5% of patients.	3
Premutation of *FRM1* gene is present in 13% of familial cases of POI.	2b
NOBOX mutation is present in 5%–7% of POI patients.	2b
More than 30 genes have been identified so far as candidate genes in human POI.	2b

TABLE 6.2

Grade of Strength for Recommendations

Recommendation	Grade Strength
In all patients, when POI is suspected, FSH should be measured twice, at least 1 month apart.	B
In all patients with POI, a karyotype should be performed.	B
In all patients with POI, an autoimmune cause of the disease should be ruled out.	B
TSH, anti-thyroid, and anti 21 hydroxylase antibodies should be measured.	B
In all patients with POI, premutation of *FMR1* gene should be searched for.	B
In all patients with POI, AMH serum level should be measured.	B
In patients with POI, NGS sequencing is able to test a panel of candidate genes.	B
Reversibility of POI is present in 4%–8% of POI women.	C
Hormone replacement therapy is necessary at least up to the age of natural menopause.	B

REFERENCES

1. De Vos M, Devroey P, Fauser BC. Primary ovarian insufficiency. Lancet. 2010; 376(9744):911–21.
2. The ESHRE guideline group on POI. ESHRE guideline: Management of women with premature ovarian insufficiency. Hum Reprod. 2016; 31:926–37.
3. Morgan S, Anderson RA, Gourley C, Wallace WH, Spears N. How do chemotherapeutic agents damage the ovary? Hum Reprod Update. 2012; 18(5):525–35.
4. Béranger R, Hoffmann P, Christin-Maitre S, Bonneterre V. Occupational exposure to chemicals as a possible etiology in premature ovarian failure: A critical analysis of the literature. Reprod Toxicol. 2012; 33:269–79.
5. Gallicchio L, Miller S, Greene T, Zacur H, Flaws JA. Premature ovarian failure among hairdressers. Hum Reprod. 2009; 24(10):2636–41.
6. Coccia ME, Rizzello F, Mariani G, Bulletti C, Palagiano A, Scarselli G. Ovarian surgery for bilateral endometriomas influences age at menopause. Hum Reprod. 2011; 26(11):3000–7.
7. Hovatta O. Ovarian function and in vitro fertilization (IVF) in Turner syndrome. Pediatr Endocrinol Rev. 2012; 9(Suppl. 2):713–7.
8. Fassnacht W, Mempel A, Strowitzki T, Vogt PH. Premature ovarian failure (POF) syndrome: Towards the molecular clinical analysis of its genetic complexity. 2006; 13(12):1397–410.
9. Rizzolio F, Pramparo T, Sala C, Zuffardi O, De Santis L, Rabellotti E. Epigenetic analysis of the critical region I for premature ovarian failure: Demonstration of a highly heterochromatic domain on the long arm of the mammalian X chromosome. J Med Genet. 2009; 46(9):585–92.
10. Perheentupa J. APS-1/APECED: The clinical disease and therapy. Endocrinol Metab Clin North Am. 2002; 31(2):295–320.
11. Reato G, Morlin L, Chen S, Furmaniak J, Smith BR, Masiero S et al. Premature ovarian failure in patients with autoimmune Addison's disease: Clinical, genetic and immunological evaluation. J Clin Endocrinol Metab. 2011; 96(8):1255–61.
12. Welt CK, Falorni A, Taylor AE, Martin KA, Hall JE. Selective theca cell dysfunction in autoimmune oophoritis results in multifollicular development, decreased estradiol, and elevated inhibin B levels. J Clin Endocrinol Metab. 2005; 90(5):3069–76.
13. La Marca A, Marzotti S, Brozzetti A, Stabile G, Artenisio AC, Bini V et al. Primary ovarian insufficiency due to steroidogenic cell autoimmunity is associated with a preserved pool of functioning follicles. J Clin Endocrinol Metab. 2009; 94(10):3816–23.
14. Grynberg M, Peltoketo H, Christin-Maitre S, Poulain M, Bouchard P, Fanchin R. First birth achieved after in vitro maturation of oocytes from a woman endowed with multiple antral follicles unresponsive to follicle-stimulating hormone. J Clin Endocrinol Metab. 2013; 98(11):4493–98.
15. Beysen D, De Paepe A, De Baere E. FOXL2 mutations and genomic rearrangements in BPES. Hum Mutat. 2009; 30(2):158–69.
16. Al Asiri S, Basit S, Wood-Trageser MA, Yatsenko SA, Jeffries EP, Surti U et al. Exome sequencing reveals MCM8 mutation underlies ovarian insufficiency and chromosomal instability. J Clin Invest. 2015; 125(1):258–62.

17. Sullivan SD, Welt S, Sherman S. FMR1 and the continuum of primary ovarian insufficiency. Semin Reprod Med. 2011; 29(4):299–307.
18. Lourenço D, Brauner R, Lin L, De Perdigo A, Weryha G, Muresan M et al. Mutations in NR5A1 associated with ovarian insufficiency. N Engl J Med. 2009; 360(12):1200–10.
19. Persani L, Rossetti R, Di Pasquale E, Cacciatore C, Fabre S. The fundamental role of bone morphogenetic protein 15 in ovarian function and its involvement in female fertility disorders. Hum Reprod Update. 2014; 20(6):869–83.
20. Bouilly J, Roucher-Boulez F, Gompel A, Bry-Gauillard H, Azibi K, Beldjord C et al. New NOBOX mutations identified in a large cohort of women with primary ovarian insufficiency decrease KIT-L expression. J Clin Endocrinol Metab. 2015; 100(3):994–1001.
21. Kasippillai T, MacArthur DG, Kirby A, Thomas B, Lambalk CB, Daly MJ, Welt CK. Mutations in eIF4ENIF1 are associated with primary ovarian insufficiency. J Clin Endocrinol Metab. 2013; 98(9):1534–9.
22. Caburet S, Arboleda VA, Llano E, Overbeek PA, Barbero JL, Oka K et al. Mutant cohesion in premature ovarian failure. N Engl J Med. 2014; 370(10):943–9.
23. Hyon C, Mansour-Hendili L, Chantot-Bastaraud S, Donadille B, Kerlan V, Dode C et al. Deletion of *CPEB1* gene: A rare but recurrent cause of premature ovarian insufficieny. J Clin Endocrinal Metab. 2016; Mar 22 jc20161291. [Epub ahead of print.]

7

Other Endocrine Disorders Causing Anovulation: Congenital Adrenal Hyperplasia

Héctor F. Escobar-Morreale and Fahrettin Keleştimur

Introduction

The congenital adrenal hyperplasias (CAH) are a group of relatively rare autosomal recessive disorders that result from mutations (in homozygosity or double heterozygosity) in the genes encoding several enzymes or proteins involved in the synthesis of adrenal steroids. They share a common pathophysiologic mechanism that consists of a deficiency in the synthesis and secretion of cortisol, the main glucocorticoid in humans. Although certain mechanisms are not completely understood, cortisol deficiency results in compensatory stimulation of the hypothalamic–pituitary axis, hypersecretion of corticotropin-releasing hormone (CRH) and corticotropin (ACTH), and hyperplasia of the dysfunctional adrenal glands (1).

The clinical presentation and consequences of CAHs depend on the gene mutated and on the degree of protein or enzymatic deficiency resulting from these mutations. Deficiency of 21α-hydroxylase accounts for approximately 90% of cases of CAH with 11β-hydroxylase deficiencies being second in frequency in most populations and 17α-hydroxylase, 3β-hydroxysteroid dehydrogenase, and steroidogenic acute response protein/20-22 desmolase deficiencies being much rarer (1). In general, the most severe forms are termed "classic CAH" and are present at birth whereas milder forms are termed "nonclassic CAH" and are diagnosed after 6 years of age. However, the genotype/phenotype concordance is not always perfect in these disorders.

All CAHs influence reproduction, either as the consequence of adrenal androgen excess (21α-hydroxylase and 11β-hydroxylase deficiencies) or as the result of a severe deficiency in the synthesis and secretion of gonadal steroids (3β-hydroxysteroid dehydrogenase, 17α-hydroxylase, and steroidogenic acute response protein/20-22 desmolase deficiencies) (LOE 2a) (1).

Patients with 3β-hydroxysteroid dehydrogenase, 17α-hydroxylase, and steroidogenic acute response protein/20-22 desmolase deficiencies present with female hypogonadism or male pseudohermaphroditism, and most patients are infertile (with the very rare exception of a few cases characterized by mild enzymatic deficiencies of 3β-hydroxysteroid dehydrogenase or 17α-hydroxylase (2,3)) (LOE 3). Hence, this chapter focuses on 21α-hydroxylase and 11β-hydroxylase deficiencies, in which adrenal androgen excess may exert a negative impact on fertility, requiring ovulation induction and/or assisted reproductive technology (4). Moreover, the presentation of nonclassic 21α-hydroxylase and 11β-hydroxylase deficiencies may be indistinguishable from functional forms of female hyperandrogenism, such as polycystic ovary syndrome or idiopathic hyperandrogenism (LOE 2a). These CAHs must be excluded before a diagnosis of functional androgen excess is made (5) at least in patients of certain ethnicity in which asymptomatic carriers of these genetic adrenal disorders are more frequent (Grade B).

Classic 21α-Hydroxylase and 11β-Hydroxylase Deficiencies

The classic form of 21α-hydroxylase deficiency is present at birth and diagnosed by neonatal screening or by clinical findings soon after birth or in early infancy, depending on the severity of the deficiency. The most severe form associates cortisol and aldosterone deficiency with severe androgen excess and is termed "salt-wasting" 21α-hydroxylase deficiency. "Simple-virilizing" 21α-hydroxylase deficiency is a milder form in which aldosterone deficiency is not clinically apparent, and androgen excess causes the symptoms. Accordingly, virilization of external genitalia at birth dominates the picture in girls whereas in boys with salt-wasting CAH, failure to thrive, dehydration, hyponatremia, and hyperkalemia typically appear within the first 2 weeks of postnatal life (6). In boys with simple-virilizing CAH that was not detected by neonatal screening, early virilization appears usually before 4 years of age (6).

In classic 11β-hydroxylase deficiency, different grades of virilization of external genitalia in girls and penile enlargement in boys are present at birth and may be followed by early sexual maturation in infancy, but instead of mineralocorticoid deficiency, these patients present with hypertension because of the increased secretion of 11-deoxycorticosterone, which is a potent mineralocorticoid (7).

Infertility is common in classic 21α-hydroxylase and 11β-hydroxylase deficiencies, and its severity parallels that of the enzymatic deficiency (LOE 2a). Sexual functioning may be impaired by anatomic distortion of external genitalia even after reconstructive surgery, delayed gender assignment, and altered psychosexual development. As a result, many female patients with classic CAH never try to conceive (4,8) (LOE 2a). Also, increased androgen concentrations leading to anovulation and increased non-cycling progesterone levels decreasing endometrium receptivity in women and inhibition of gonadotropin secretion and testicular adrenal rest tumors that may obstruct seminiferous tubules in men (4,8) may contribute to infertility (LOE 2b).

Patients with classic CAH seeking fertility usually require intensification of their adrenal steroid replacement therapy (with glucocorticoids and in salt-wasting forms with gluco- and mineralocorticoids) with the aim of suppressing androgen and progesterone excess (to below 2 nmol/l), and reducing testicular rest tumors in men (4,8,9) (Grade B). The latter might require surgery, but the results toward restoration of fertility are uncertain (8). Intensification of replacement therapy in women with classic CAH results in pregnancy rates comparable to that of the normal population, yet the fertility rates are much lower (9) (LOE 2b). However, a significant number of women with classic CAH require ovulation induction or assisted reproductive technology to conceive (4) (LOE 2a). As in other causes of adrenal insufficiency, women with classic CAH may need stress glucocorticoid regimens during delivery of surgery.

Nonclassic 21α-Hydroxylase and 11β-Hydroxylase Deficiencies

In these milder forms of CAH, salt-wasting (in 21α-hydroxylase deficiency) and hypertension (in 11β-hydroxylase deficiency) are absent, and the clinical course is similar to that of other causes of functional androgen excess (LOE 2a). The phenotype of nonclassic 21α-hydroxylase deficiency resembles that of nonclassic 11β-hydroxylase deficiency. Girls and boys may present after 6 years of age with mild symptoms of androgen excess, such as moderately accelerated growth velocity or premature adrenarche, but most cases are diagnosed after puberty when girls may present with symptoms indistinguishable from those of polycystic ovary syndrome, such as hirsutism or menstrual dysfunction (8). Moreover, there are cryptic cases in which no symptoms are present and which are diagnosed in the context of familial studies.

Fertility is not severely compromised in nonclassic CAH, and many patients conceive spontaneously because ovulation may not be compromised, and testicular adrenal rest tumors are exceptional in this population (4) (LOE 2b). Glucocorticoids are not needed in patients with nonclassic CAH during adulthood if symptoms are absent. Hyperandrogenic symptoms should be managed with oral contraceptives or anti-androgens because, as occurs in patients with polycystic ovary syndrome, glucocorticoids rarely provide adequate control of hirsutism and acne. However, glucocorticoid administration with the aim of reducing androgen and progesterone concentrations may be useful in women trying to conceive in order to restore ovulation and facilitate implantation (4) (Grade B). Single oral doses as low as 1.25–2.5 mg of prednisone at nighttime may be useful in this regard. If glucocorticoid replacement is not useful in restoring ovulation after a few months, clomiphene or gonadotropins can be used (LOE 2b). As opposed to women with classic CAH, patients with nonclassic CAH do not need any special attention during pregnancy or delivery.

Genetic Counseling and Prenatal Treatment for At-Risk Pregnancies

Genetic counseling should be offered to patients with classic and nonclassic CAH (Grade B). Carrier frequencies for alleles causing classic 21α-hydroxylase deficiency are approximately 1:60, and the risk of a patient with classic 21α-hydroxylase deficiency of having a child with classic CAH is 1:20 (4) (LOE 2a). Moreover, women with nonclassic 21α-hydroxylase deficiency may give birth to a fetus affected with classic 21α-hydroxylase deficiency [with frequencies as high as 2.5% in some series (10)] because nonclassic patients frequently are compound heterozygotes for mild and severe mutations (LOE 2b). Genetic counseling is crucial for patients at-risk of having a child with classic CAH because of the following reasons:

* Experimental prenatal treatment with exogenous dexamethasone may prevent virilization of affected female fetuses in approximately 80%–85% of cases (LOE 2b). However, this treatment is currently being questioned because dexamethasone may have significant maternal and fetal side effects (LOE 2a). Fetal sex determination by detection of the Y chromosome in males in the maternal serum (SRY test) may be useful to avoid prenatal dexamethasone in males (11) (Grade C). If any, such a therapeutic approach should be restricted to centers with experience that apply protocols approved by institutional review boards (8) (Grade B).
* Nowadays, assisted reproductive technology permits preimplantation genetic diagnosis and avoidance of the transfer of affected embryos resulting from IVF (4) (Grade D).

Conclusions

CAHs are rare disorders that may exert a negative impact on fertility, especially in the more severe classic forms (LOE 2a). Intensification of replacement therapy with gluco- and mineralocorticoids may improve pregnancy rates in women with classic CAH (LOE 2a), and glucocorticoid treatment may facilitate pregnancy in women with nonclassic CAH (LOE 2b). Ovulation induction and assisted reproductive technology may be helpful when this approach fails (LOE 2a and 2b for classic and nonclassic CAH). The milder nonclassic forms of 21α-hydroxylase and 11β-hydroxylase deficiencies are indistinguishable from other forms of class II oligo-ovulation and must be ruled out in certain populations because they carry a significant risk for having a child affected by classic CAH (Grade B). Genetic counseling should be offered to all patients with CAH, irrespective of the severity of their disease (Grade B).

TABLE 7.1

Level of Evidence of Statements

Statement	Level of Evidence
CAHs influence reproduction, either as the consequence of adrenal androgen excess or as the result of a severe deficiency in the synthesis and secretion of gonadal steroids.	2a
Patients with 3β-hydroxysteroid dehydrogenase, 17α-hydroxylase, and steroidogenic acute response protein/20-22 desmolase deficiencies present with female hypogonadism or male pseudohermaphroditism, and most are infertile.	3
The presentation of nonclassic CAH may be indistinguishable from functional forms of female hyperandrogenism.	2a
Infertility is common in classic CAH, and its severity parallels that of the enzymatic deficiency.	2a
Many women with classic CAH never try to conceive.	2a
Increased androgen concentrations and increased non-cycling progesterone levels in women and inhibition of gonadotropin secretion and testicular adrenal rest tumors in men may contribute to infertility.	2b
Intensification of replacement therapy in women with classic CAH results in pregnancy rates comparable to that of the normal population, yet the fertility rates are much lower.	2b
A significant number of women with classic CAH require ovulation induction or assisted reproductive technology to conceive.	2a
Fertility is not severely compromised in nonclassic CAH, and many patients conceive spontaneously.	2b
If glucocorticoid replacement is not useful in restoring ovulation in women with nonclassic CAH, clomiphene or gonadotropins can be used.	2b
Carrier frequencies for alleles causing classic 21α-hydroxylase deficiency are approximately 1:60, and the risk of a patient with classic 21α-hydroxylase deficiency of having a child with classic CAH is 1:20.	2a
Women with nonclassic 21α-hydroxylase deficiency may give birth to a fetus affected with classic 21α-hydroxylase deficiency because they frequently are compound heterozygotes for mild and severe mutations.	2b
Experimental prenatal treatment with exogenous dexamethasone may prevent virilization of affected female fetuses in approximately 80%–85% of cases.	2b
This treatment is currently being questioned because dexamethasone may have significant maternal and fetal side effects.	2a

TABLE 7.2

Grade of Strength for Recommendations

Recommendation	Grade Strength
Nonclassic forms of 21α-hydroxylase and 11β-hydroxylase deficiencies are indistinguishable from other forms of class II oligoovulation and must be ruled out in certain populations because they carry a significant risk for having a child affected by classic CAH.	B
Patients with classic CAH seeking fertility usually require intensification of their adrenal steroid replacement therapy with the aim of suppressing androgen and progesterone excess and reducing testicular rest tumors in men.	B
Glucocorticoid replacement should be offered to women with nonclassic CAH trying to conceive.	B
Genetic counseling should be offered to patients with classic and nonclassic CAH.	B
Fetal sex determination by detection of the Y chromosome in males in the maternal serum (SRY test) may be useful to avoid prenatal dexamethasone in males.	C
Assisted reproductive technology permits preimplantation genetic diagnosis and avoidance of the transfer of affected embryos resulting from IVF.	D

REFERENCES

1. Nieman LK. Adrenal steroid biosynthesis. Philadelphia: Wolters Kluwer; 2012.

2. Alos N, Moisan AM, Ward L, Desrochers M, Legault L, Leboeuf G et al. A novel A10E homozygous mutation in the HSD3B2 gene causing severe salt-wasting 3beta-hydroxysteroid dehydrogenase deficiency in 46,XX and 46,XY French-Canadians: Evaluation of gonadal function after puberty. J Clin Endocrinol Metab. 2000 May; 85(5):1968–74.

3. Levran D, Ben-Shlomo I, Pariente C, Dor J, Mashiach S, Weissman A. Familial partial 17,20-desmolase and 17alpha-hydroxylase deficiency presenting as infertility. J Assist Reprod Genet. 2003 Jan; 20(1):21–8.

4. Reichman DE, White PC, New MI, Rosenwaks Z. Fertility in patients with congenital adrenal hyperplasia. Fertil Steril. 2014 Feb; 101(2):301–9.

5. Azziz R. Controversy in clinical endocrinology: Diagnosis of polycystic ovarian syndrome: The Rotterdam criteria are premature. J Clin Endocrinol Metab. 2006 Mar; 91(3):781–5.

6. Merke DP. Genetics and clinical presentation of classic congenital adrenal hyperplasia due to 21-hydroxylase deficiency. Philadelphia: Wolters Kluwer; 2013.

7. Nieman LK. Congenital adrenal hyperplasia due to 11-beta-hydroxylase deficiency. Philadelphia: Wolters Kluwer; 2014.

8. Speiser PW, Azziz R, Baskin LS, Ghizzoni L, Hensle TW, Merke DP et al. Congenital adrenal hyperplasia due to steroid 21-hydroxylase deficiency: An Endocrine Society clinical practice guideline. J Clin Endocrinol Metab. 2010 Sep; 95(9):4133–60.

9. Casteras A, De Silva P, Rumsby G, Conway GS. Reassessing fecundity in women with classical congenital adrenal hyperplasia (CAH): Normal pregnancy rate but reduced fertility rate. Clin Endocrinol (Oxf). 2009 Jun; 70(6):833–7.

10. Moran C, Azziz R, Weintrob N, Witchel SF, Rohmer V, Dewailly D et al. Reproductive outcome of women with 21-hydroxylase-deficient nonclassic adrenal hyperplasia. J Clin Endocrinol Metab. 2006 Sep; 91(9):3451–6.

11. Tardy-Guidollet V, Menassa R, Costa JM, David M, Bouvattier-Morel C, Baumann C et al. New management strategy of pregnancies at risk of congenital adrenal hyperplasia using fetal sex determination in maternal serum: French cohort of 258 cases (2002–2011). J Clin Endocrinol Metab. 2014 Apr; 99(4):1180–8.

8

Other Endocrine Disorders Causing Anovulation: Thyroid Disorders

Alex F. Muller

Introduction

Thyroid dysfunction has profound effects on the chance of becoming and remaining pregnant (1). Hyperthyroidism as well as hypothyroidism is associated with irregular menstrual cycles. Similarly, thyroid dysfunction interferes with normal fertility, and hence, it is associated with subfertility. Moreover, relevant data point to an important role for thyroid hormone in the earliest phases of pregnancy with the well-described syndrome of cretinism on the one end of the spectrum and the less well-described syndrome of maternal hypothyroxinaemia on the other end of the spectrum (2). For the aim of the current chapter, it is important to point out that even small changes in thyroid hormone levels—such as can be induced by ovarian hyperstimulation (vide infra)—are already associated with impaired psychomotor development in the offspring.

During pregnancy, thyroid hormone metabolism changes in a well-characterized manner (2). There is quite a bit of literature on the physiological changes in thyroid hormone metabolism during normal pregnancy, and for an in-depth review on this topic, the reader is referred to the existing literature (2); however, in order to provide a better understanding, a short review of the normal response of the thyroid to pregnancy will be given first. Then, changes in thyroid function induced by ovulation induction will be discussed followed by an overview of how thyroid dysfunction will affect the results of ovulation induction. Finally, we will try to make some recommendations on what to advise women undergoing ovulation induction.

Thyroid Function and Becoming Pregnant

Menstrual disturbances are associated with thyrotoxicosis and hypothyroidism (1). The prevalence of menstrual disturbances in thyrotoxicosis varies between 22% and 65% and in hypothyroidism between 23% and 80%, with the lower prevalences reported in the more recent studies (1). Treatment of hypothyroidism reduces the prevalence of menstrual disturbances to the normal population level (1). The changes in menstrual cycle are due to changes in estrogens, androgens, gonadotrophins, and sex-hormone binding globulin (1).

Fertility—that is, the ability to conceive after 1 year of regular and unprotected intercourse—is generally thought to be negatively influenced by thyroid dysfunction. It should be noted, however, that the studies on fertility in women with thyroid dysfunction are mostly observational, uncontrolled, and retrospective.

Subclinical hypothyroidism is associated with subfertility: Women with higher TSHs have lower pregnancy rates and take longer to become pregnant (LOE 3). Moreover, thyroid hormone substitution improves the chances of becoming pregnant (1) (LOE 3). Considering overt hypothyroidism, there are only limited data; however, in analyzing menstrual disturbances or infertility, a TSH—and subsequent fT4 if it is outside the reference range—determination is indicated, and in case of overt hypothyroidism, treatment with thyroid hormone substitution is indicated (LOE 4) (1).

In a prospective study, thyrotoxicosis was not more prevalent in infertile women compared to controls (1). Data from older studies suggest that women with overt hyperthyroidism remain ovulatory, albeit with a higher prevalence of menstrual disturbances (1).

Thyroid autoimmunity—that is, the presence of thyroid peroxidase (TPO) and/or thyroglobulin (Tg) antibodies—is also associated with impaired fertility, suggesting a common immunological background for thyroid dysfunction and infertility (1). This notion is supported by the fact that the chances of a miscarriage are approximately doubled in euthyroid women with thyroid antibodies (1). This was investigated in 77 women with a normal thyroid function and without thyroid autoimmunity prior to their first assisted reproductive technology procedure; of these women, 32 suffered a miscarriage. In the women who suffered a miscarriage and in the ones with ongoing pregnancy, thyroid function changed significantly, but these changes were not different between those with ongoing pregnancies and those with a miscarriage (1) (LOE 2a).

Taken together, we can conclude that both hypo- and hyperthyroidism are associated with cycle disturbances. With respect to fertility, the data are less clear. Although not supported by high-quality intervention studies, treatment of subclinical hypothyroidism and overt hypothyroidism (i.e., a TSH level above the reference range) is advised as an attempt to restore fertility. Overt thyrotoxicosis should be treated, but clear data showing the extent of such an intervention on menstrual cycle and fertility are lacking.

Thyroid Function during Pregnancy

Several mechanisms are at play during pregnancy that lead to physiological changes in thyroid hormone metabolism (2).

First, hCG has a structural homology with TSH, and the rise of hCG in the first trimester of pregnancy leads to an increase in fT4 and a suppression in TSH. Second, estradiol results in a rise in TBG and therefore TT4, leading to a fall in fT4, resulting in a compensatory rise in TSH, so more thyroid hormones are produced, and a new steady state will ensue. Third, during pregnancy, fluid retention leads to a larger distribution volume of thyroxin, which needs to be compensated by the production of extra thyroid hormones. Fourth, there is transport of thyroid hormone from the mother to the fetus.

So the hormonal changes during pregnancy collectively lead to an increased requirement of thyroid hormones in order to maintain euthyroidism.

Women who are on thyroid hormone replacement need to increase their thyroxine dosage during pregnancy in order to remain euthyroid. Determination of TSH-receptor antibodies is only indicated in women who are hypothyroid as a result of prior treatment of Graves' disease.

Thyroid Function and Ovulation Induction

Clomiphene Citrate

As clomiphene citrate leads to a rise in FSH concentration of about 50% with a subsequent rise in estradiol production, some influence—a temporary lowering of fT4 concentration—on thyroid hormone levels is to be expected. In a small study ($n = 8$), the presence of TPO-antibodies was associated with a poor treatment response to clomiphene citrate in women with PCOS, which might be taken to suggest that a reduced thyroid hormone reserve in these women led to a poor response to clomiphene (LOE 3). However, in another study in euthyroid women with functional hypothalamic amenorrhea, administration of L-thyroxine did not improve the response to clomiphene citrate with respect to the number of ovulatory cycles or luteal phase defects (LOE 2b). Unfortunately, these studies are small, and the study populations differ. Thus, no clear conclusion can be drawn on the influence the thyroid hormone status has on the effect of clomiphene citrate, or vice versa.

Tamoxifen

The data on tamoxifen and thyroid function are generated from older studies in postmenopausal women with breast cancer, so the question remains whether these data are also true for premenopausal women who use this agent in the setting of ovulation induction. In all these studies, TBG increased with a concomitant rise in total T4 (LOE 3). In one study from Norway in which 26 postmenopausal women with breast cancer were treated with tamoxifen, fT4 concentrations fell, and TSH rose (LOE 3). In two other studies collectively studying 87 women with breast cancer, fT4 levels remained stable over a treatment period of 6 months (LOE 3). In one of these studies, a significant increase of TSH was noted at the end of 3 months with a subsequent decrease at the end of 6 months whereas in the other study basal as well as TRH-stimulated TSH increased significantly after tamoxifen treatment. These variations in thyroid hormone dynamics could reflect differences in iodine supply in the areas where these studies were done; unfortunately, no data were given on thyroid autoantibodies.

Taken together, it seems safe to say that tamoxifen—at least in the context of breast cancer treatment in postmenopausal women—leads to a rise in TBG and, therefore, leads to an increased demand on the thyroid as reflected by a rise in TSH.

Gonadotrophin Therapy

From 2000 onward, several studies have been performed to investigate the impact of ovarian hyperstimulation on thyroid function. In 65 Dutch women who underwent controlled ovarian hyperstimulation, fT4 decreased with a concomitant rise in TSH (3) (LOE 3). In the same time span, estradiol and TBG increased, supporting the proposed mechanism whereby ovarian hyperstimulation leads to hyperestrogenism, which, in turn, leads to increased TBG levels and, therefore, a decrease in fT4 with a concomitant rise in TSH. In another study from Brussels, Belgium, the changes in thyroid hormone levels after controlled ovarian hyperstimulation were followed until the end of the first trimester (1) (LOE 3). Also in this study, the role of thyroid autoimmunity was further investigated. Thirty-five women who became pregnant after controlled ovarian hyperstimulation—nine of which had thyroid autoantibodies—were studied before and during the first trimester of pregnancy. In this study, both TSH and fT4 rose significantly during controlled ovarian hyperstimulation (1). Interestingly, patterns of serum TSH and fT4 changes were different over time in TPO-antibody positive versus negative participants with higher TSH and lower fT4 levels in the TPO-positive women (1).

In another study, the changes in thyroid function during different regimens of ovarian hyperstimulation were studied and compared with the normal menstrual cycle. A total of 97 women were studied: 20 underwent intrauterine insemination in a natural cycle, 27 underwent intrauterine insemination with mild ovarian hyperstimulation, and 50 underwent in vitro fertilization. In this study, again, there was a clear relationship between estradiol and TBG on the one hand and TBG and fT4 on the other hand. Midluteal estradiol, TBG, and total T4 concentrations were higher, and fT4 concentrations lower in ovarian hyperstimulation compared to natural cycle. Women in the in vitro fertilization group showed the highest estradiol levels and the lowest fT4 levels during the midluteal phase. Interestingly, these women had the lowest TSH levels at baseline, which rose during the midluteal phase. Unfortunately, no thyroid antibodies were determined in this study, so the possible contribution of thyroid autoimmunity in these changes is unknown (4) (LOE 3).

In a retrospective analysis, the effects of ovarian hyperstimulation syndrome have been investigated; 52 women with uncomplicated ovarian hyperstimulation were compared with 25 women who developed ovarian hyperstimulation syndrome. Despite higher estradiol levels in those with ovarian hyperstimulation syndrome compared to those without the syndrome, no significant differences in the changes in thyroid function were observed (LOE 3). This is most likely due to the opposing effects of estradiol (ultimately leading to a lowering in fT4) and hCG with an intrinsic thyrotropic action (1).

All these studies are only partially concordant, indicating the need for further study. But what is clear from all these studies is that ovulation induction with gonadotrophins has a lowering effect on fT4 levels, and especially in the presence of thyroid autoimmunity, this may even lead to subclinical hypothyroidism during pregnancy.

Discussion

Relevant data show that, both for becoming pregnant as well as remaining pregnant, a normal thyroid function is important. In women with hypothyroidism and thyrotoxicosis, and possibly even in euthyroid women with thyroid autoimmunity, there is an increased frequency of various adverse pregnancy outcomes (miscarriage, preterm delivery, impaired psychomotor development in the offspring, preeclampsia, stillbirth, congestive heart failure, thyroid storm). So it is clear that overt thyroid function disorders need to be treated (1) (LOE 3).

Before 10 to 12 weeks gestation, the fetal brain is fully dependent on the maternal supply of thyroid hormone, and high levels of TSH—and even low normal fT4 levels—have been associated with impaired cognitive development in the offspring. Therefore, assisted reproduction gives us an opportunity to determine the thyroid status prior to the period in which the fetal brain is most dependent on an adequate supply of maternal thyroid hormone. Thus in light of the described effects of ovulation induction (further lowering of fT4), subclinical hypothyroidism should be treated with thyroxin aiming for a TSH below 2.5 mU/L (5) (LOE 4).

Regarding the issue of thyroid autoimmunity in otherwise euthyroid women, it is at present unclear what to do other than to monitor thyroid function (as thyroid autoimmunity poses a risk factor for development of hypothyroidism).

Conclusions

Thyroid dysfunction is associated with cycle disturbances and reduced fertility. Ovulation induction has a lowering effect of fT4. In infertile women with subclinical hypothyroidism, indirect evidence suggests that treatment aiming for TSH below 2.5 mU/L is beneficial (5). In women with thyroid antibodies (but with a normal TSH) it seems reasonable to aim for TSH below 2.5 mU/L as well.

TABLE 8.1

Level of Evidence of Statements

Statement	Level of Evidence
Thyroid dysfunction is associated with menstrual disturbances.	3
Treatment of thyroid dysfunction will restore menstrual cyclicity.	2b
Ovulation induction with clomiphene citrate and tamoxifen has uncertain effects on thyroid function.	4
Ovulation induction with gonadotrophins leads to a lowering in fT4 in women with thyroid autoimmunity.	1b

TABLE 8.2

Grade of Strength for Recommendations

Recommendation	Grade Strength
Overt hypothyroidism and overt thyrotoxicosis should be treated in women desiring to become pregnant.	D
Subclinical hypothyroidism should be treated in women desiring to become pregnant with the aim of a TSH below 2.5 mU/L.	B

REFERENCES

1. Krassas GE, Poppe K, Glinoer D. Thyroid function and human reproductive health. Endocr Rev. 2010 Oct; 31(5):702–55.
2. Glinoer D. The regulation of thyroid function in pregnancy: Pathways of endocrine adaptation from physiology to pathology. Endocr Rev. 1997 Jun; 18(3):404–33.
3. Muller AF, Verhoeff A, Mantel MJ, De Jong FH, Berghout A. Decrease of free thyroxine levels after controlled ovarian hyperstimulation. J Clin Endocrinol Metab. 2000 Feb; 85(2):545–8.
4. Fleischer KM, Muller AF, Hohmann FP, de Jong F, Eijkemans MJC, Fauser BC, Laven JSE. Impact of controlled ovarian hyperstimulation on thyroid function. Reproductive Biology Insights. 2014; 7:9–16.
5. Velkeniers B, Van Meerhaeghe A, Poppe K, Unuane D, Tournaye H, Haentjens P. Levothyroxine treatment and pregnancy outcome in women with subclinical hypothyroidism undergoing assisted reproduction technologies: Systematic review and meta-analysis of RCTs. Hum Reprod Update. 2013 May–Jun; 19(3):251–8.

9

Other Endocrine Disorders Causing Anovulation: Prolactinomas

Sebastian J. C. M. M. Neggers and Aart J. van der Lely*†

Introduction

Prolactin (PRL) plays an essential role in post-mating reproductive functions in many species. Obvious examples are lactation, metabolic adaptations, migrations, behavioral adaptations (broodiness, suppression of aggression), and (seasonal) gonadal suppression (1,2). From this perspective, PRL is the reproductive hormone that takes over where the gonadotropins leave off, driving reproductive functions that are segregated, both in time and type, from those of the pre-mating phase (3).

Lactotroph cells of the anterior pituitary gland produce PRL. Hypothalamic neurons release dopamine that has an inhibitory control over the PRL production. PRL directly regulates its own secretion as well via the hypothalamus. Classical stimulation of the PRL secretion occurs during suckling of the nipples during breastfeeding directly via the hypothalamus and pituitary gland (4). During early gestation, the corpus luteum is supported by high serum levels of PRL (5). PRL also has an immunomodulatory function, increasing IL-12 and IL-10 production and the regulating cytokine profile (6). During gestation, elevated PRL levels are tied to elevated estrogen levels, together with increased PRL receptor expression in the hypothalamus (7), suggesting that the hypothalamus has an increased sensitivity for PRL. The human placenta produces increasing amounts of placental lactogen (hPL) during gestation (8). HPL has a similar molecular structural to PRL and can bind to PRL receptors. HPL is not regulated by the hypothalamic dopamine neurons. HPL levels peak mid-gestation and are predominantly secreted into the amniotic fluid and in fetal and maternal body fluids, including cerebrospinal fluid. So, in human gestation, a major increase in both PRL and placental hPL have been observed (9).

Patholophysiology

One of the most common neuro-endocrine abnormalities is prolactin hypersecretion due to pituitary–hypothalamic disorders. Lactotroph adenomas (prolactinomas) are the most frequent secreting pituitary adenomas. Usually, surgery and medical therapy are the cornerstones of pituitary adenoma treatment. However, lactotroph adenomas are a notable exception as medical therapy is the only treatment of choice in virtually all patients.

Hyperprolactinemia by itself is not exclusively caused by lactotroph adenomas and may also occur as a result of using several types of medication, some systemic disorders, and sometimes other pituitary adenomas. In general, pituitary adenomas should be treated by a multidisciplinary team, in which

* SN received research grants and speakers fees from Ipsen and Pfizer.
† AvdL consultant and received speakers fees from Novartis, Ipsen, and Pfizer.

different specialties closely collaborate: (neuro)endocrinologists, neurosurgeons, ENT-surgeons, neuro-radiologists, ophthalmologists, and radiotherapists. Microprolactinomas (adenoma size <1 cm) are probably the exception to the general rule that pituitary adenomas should be treated in a multidisciplinary fashion. However, incidentalomas are commonly observed on pituitary magnetic resonance images (MRIs), ranging from 10%–38% (10,11). Therefore, it can be difficult to distinguish hyperprolactinemia due to other causes than a prolactinoma from hyperprolactinemia due to a small prolactinoma. Neuro-endocrinologists are used to address this diagnostic riddle in pituitary disorders. In this chapter, we discuss (patho)physiology, diagnostic strategy, and treatment options.

Hyperprolactinemia

Symptoms

Galactorrhea (12) and gonadal dysfunction are common symptoms of hyperprolactinemia in women, but galactorrhea is very rare in men and postmenopausal women as the low estrogen (E2) state of men and postmenopausal women protects them against galactorrhea. Galactorrhea can occur in different forms, such as transient, alternating, spontaneous, and upon breast manipulation.

Women

Hyperprolactinemia is the cause of amenorrhea in about 10%–20% of cases, provided that pregnancy is excluded. Often, gonadotropin levels are within the normal ranges but can be decreased, which results in hypogonadism. Hyperprolactinemia inhibits the gonadal axis by decreasing the release of gonadotrophin-releasing hormone (GnRH). This drop in GnRH results in a decreased release of luteinizing hormone (LH) and, to a lesser extent, follicle-stimulating hormone (FSH). The magnitude of the increased prolactin serum levels correlates with the severity of the hypogonadotropic hypogonadism and, therefore, with the severity of the symptomatology.

Men

The hypogonadotropic hypogonadism state is present in men as well and might cause symptoms such as infertility, impotence, gynecomastia, decreased libido, and decreased energy level. Contrary to women, the magnitude of hyperprolactinemia is not closely correlated with symptomatology.

Diagnosis of Hyperprolactinemia

PRL levels should be assessed whenever symptoms or a cluster of symptoms as discussed above are present. Normal levels of PRL are usually below 20 (male) to 25 (female) mcg/L. In case of mild elevations in prolactin levels (25–40 mcg/L), it is recommended to reassess prolactin before the diagnosis of hyperprolactinemia can be established. In general, a single prolactin assessment is sufficient. In Table 9.3, possible causes of hyperprolactinemia are depicted. Depending on the prolactin assay that is used, different normal ranges are used in clinical practice.

A possible pitfall in the diagnosis of hyperprolactinemia is a decreased clearance of PRL. During chronic renal failure, PRL levels are generally increased up to about three times the upper limit of normal (ULN). Another cause of hyperprolactinemia due to a decreased clearance is macroprolactinemia, which is a large aggregate of prolactin and immunoglobulin-G. When PRL levels are mildly elevated without significant symptomatology, macroprolactinemia might be a possible explanation of the high prolactin levels as reported by the lab. In symptomatic patients, however, screening for macroprolactinemia is redundant (13).

In the past, falsely low prolactin levels were reported by old assays in samples with extremely high serum levels of PRL. This phenomenon was called the "high-dose hook effect" (14) and reflects the interference with the high PRL levels in the sample and the soluble antibody of the assay. With the current

TABLE 9.3

Causes of Hyperprolactinemia

	Cause	Additional Information
Physiologic	Nipple/breast stimulation	
	Stress	
	Breastfeeding	
	Exercise	
	Sleep	
	High-protein food	
	Pregnancy	
Pathologic	Prolactinoma	
	Pituitary/hypothalamic and stalk lesions	Trauma, radiation, infiltrative disease, tumors
	Hypothyroidism	
	Trauma	
	Chronic renal failure	
	Injury to the chest wall	Like burns, trauma
Medication	Antipsychotics	First-generation drugs such as Chlorpromazine, Fluphenazine, Haloperidol
		Second-generation drugs such as Asenapine, Paliperidone, Risperidone
	Antidepressants	(Tri/tertra)cyclic antidepressants, such as Clomipramine, Monoamine oxidase inhibitors, and, to a lesser extent, selective serotonin reuptake inhibitors
	Antihypertensives	Like methyldopa, verapamil
	Gastrointestinal/antiemetics	Like metoclopramide, domperidone
	Opiates	
	Estrogen	
Other	Genetic, germ line	Familial hyperprolactinemia
	Cocaine	

modern immunoassays, however, this effect is rare although, when PRL levels are unexpectedly low in relation to the large size of a lactotroph adenoma, one should exclude this hook effect by reassessing the sample in a 1:100 dilution (13).

Diagnostic Strategies

In general, PRL levels greater than five times ULN are due to the existence of a prolactinoma. Medications that induce hyperprolactinemia rarely induce hyperprolactinemia that exceeds five times ULN. The elevated PRL levels due to the use of anti-dopaminergic medication will practically always normalize when medication is stopped. PRL concentrations between five and 15 times ULN can be due to the presence of a true prolactinoma but also can be due to the existence of other types of pituitary adenomas, infiltrative diseases, craniopharyngiomas, and other lesions in the pituitary hypothalamic region (see below for further explanation). In these cases, MRI evaluation is necessary. When no cause of hyperprolactinemia can be found, the name "idiopathic" hyperprolactinemia is used. In one third of patients with idiopathic hyperprolactinemia, PRL levels normalize spontaneously, and in 50% of them, PRL levels do not change (15,16). In a study on idiopathic hyperprolactinemia, 10% of patients developed a detectable tumor on CT/MRI after a follow up of 6 years (16). A systematic overview is depicted in Figure 9.1.

Other pituitary adenomas can be divided into two groups. One group actually co-secretes PRL together with another anterior pituitary hormone. Examples are growth hormone (GH) and/or thyrotropin stimulating hormone (TSH). Co-secreting pituitary adenomas are also called mixed tumors.

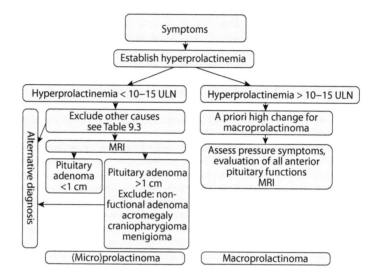

FIGURE 9.1 Systematic approach to diagnose the cause of hyperprolactinemia.

When GH and PRL are co-secreted, these tumors are called somato-lactotrophe adenoma, causing acromegaly. The combination of TSH and prolactin is called thyro-lactotrophe adenoma, causing secondary hyperthyroidism. Combinations of GH, TSH, and prolactin are very rare but also do exist.

The second group of tumors that can induce hyperprolactinemia are tumors that cause mass effects in the sellar region, resulting in a deviation or compression of the pituitary stalk. This will inhibit dopamine from the hypothalamus to reach the PRL-producing cells in the pituitary, in which dopamine decreases PRL secretion. Mass effects generally do not increase prolactin levels above 10 ULN (17). Examples of these macroadenomas (≥1 cm) are non-functioning pituitary adenomas (NFA), secreting pituitary adenomas such as GH, TSH, and, seldomly, corticotropine (ACTH). Tumors from non-pituitary origin are craniopharyngiomas, meningiomas, metastatic lesions, primary brain tumors, germ cell tumors, and infiltrating diseases such as sarcoidosis, histiocystosis, and tuberculosis.

Hyperprolactinemia of more than 10–15 times ULN is almost always caused by a macroprolactinoma (adenoma size ≥1 cm), and MRI evaluation is necessary. In the large pituitary tumors, including prolactinomas, there is a risk of developing visual field defects and sometimes the impingement of the optic chiasms that results in a loss in visual acuity. These tumors can even compress other cranial nerves, which can cause eye movement disorders and diplopia.

Treatment Focused on the Most Relevant Pituitary Adenomas Causing Hyperprolactinemia

Non-Functional Adenoma

NFA constitute about 80% of the pituitary adenomas. NFA's secretory products usually do not cause a clear recognizable syndrome and therefore are called non-functioning adenomas. Patients with an NFA seek medical attention when the adenoma size causes pressure symptoms on surrounding tissues, such as the optic chiasm, and, therefore, give rise to symptoms as headaches, visual field defects, diplopia, and symptoms related to hypopituitarism. However, the tumor mass effects can cause hypogonadism and hyperprolactinemia and mimic a prolactinoma. The treatment of choice for NFA is surgery or, if possible, a wait-and-scan policy and, in some cases, medical treatment with dopamine agonists. However, symptomatic treatment of hyperprolactinemia in NFA can be useful.

Prolactinomas

Lactotroph adenomas are the most common secreting adenomas. Adenoma size and serum PRL levels are generally correlated. Most prolactinoma patients have a PRL level higher than 200 µg/L (10 times ULN). Prolactinomas are almost exclusively treated with primary medical treatment. To date, dopamine agonists are the first line treatment as they usually rapidly normalize PRL levels and reverse galactorrhea, restore fertility, and also cause tumor shrinkage in most patients (18). In microprolactinomas, treatment is not mandatory because they rarely develop into macroprolactinomas (15,19). However, when patients seek medical attention because of symptoms, such as hypogonadism, infertility, gynecomastia, and galactorrhea, or when there is growth of the microadenoma, medical treatment is indicated. In macroprolactinomas, treatment is almost always mandatory.

In a minority of patients, other treatment modalities should be considered. Examples are prolactinomas that are resistant to dopamine agonist therapy or when the patient does not tolerate medication. In resistant prolactinomas, increasing the dose of dopamine agonists, surgery, and/or radiotherapy can be necessary. The existence of resistance to dopaminergic drugs is empirically defined. The most commonly used definition is a failure to achieve normal PRL serum levels and/or a significant reduction of tumor volume during dopamine agonist treatment (20,21).

Medical Treatment

The lactotroph adenoma cells express dopamine receptors (D1 & D2 subtypes of dopamine receptors). By binding to these D1 & D2 receptors, dopamine agonists, reduce synthesis and secretion of PRL and reduce adenoma cell size (18). In patients, dopamine agonists reduce tumor size and decrease PRL hypersecretion by the lactotroph adenoma in more than 90% of the cases. The decrease in serum PRL levels is generally accompanied by a reduction in tumor size. Within 2–3 weeks after initiation of pharmacological treatment, PRL levels tend to decrease preceding the reduction in adenoma size. After 6 weeks to 6 months of dopamine agonist treatment, a reduction in adenoma size can be observed on MRI (22). In general, the magnitude of decrease in serum prolactin levels correlates well with the decrease in tumor size (13). Finally, during dopamine agonist treatment, the decrease in hyperprolactinemia is accompanied by a reduction in signs and symptoms.

Several dopamine agonists are available for the treatment of hyperprolactinemia and prolactinomas. Depending on the patients' characteristics, therapeutic expectations, and possible side effects, the most optimal dopamine agonist should be chosen to increase efficacy and patients' compliance (23). For 30 years, bromocriptine has been used, and it is one of the oldest ergot derivatives currently available. For an optimal therapeutic effect, a twice-daily dose is necessary (24). Once or twice weekly dosing is possible with another ergot dopamine agonist cabergoline. Cabergoline is a more effective medical treatment with a lower tendency to cause nausea than bromocriptine (18,25). An ergot derivative primarily used in high doses of >3 mg/day for the treatment of Parkinson's disease is pergolide (26). Typical doses in prolactinoma patients range from 0.05 to 1.0 mg/day. Increased risk of valvular heart disease is associated with the use of high doses of pergolide for the treatment of Parkinson's disease (27). For this reason, pergolide was withdrawn from the U.S. market in 2007. Valvular heart disease is associated with high doses of a specific class of dopamine agonist, the ergot derivatives.

A non-ergot dopamine agonist, quinagolide, is registered for once daily use. The problem is that quinagolide is not available in some countries (28,29).

Efficacy of Dopamine Agonists

Cabergoline seems to be superior to bromocriptine in decreasing serum PRL levels (18). Normalization of PRL levels with an efficacy rate of 80%–90% can be expected during cabergoline treatment. A higher efficacy rate of >95% was observed when patients were up-titrated in cabergoline doses up to weekly 12 mg (30). In most studies, weekly doses over 3.5 mg are relatively rare.

Quinagolide has more or less the same efficacy as cabergoline although a few studies suggest the superiority of cabergoline (29). The great advantage is the non-ergot nature of the drug. This would imply an absence of the increased reported risk of the development of valvular heart disease, which can be seen during high-dose ergot derivate treatment.

Withdrawal of Dopamine Agonists

Remission rates after discontinuation of dopamine agonists differ significantly between studies. For macroadenomas, rates of 16%–64% and, for microadenomas, rates of 21%–69% are reported. In a recent meta-analysis, an average remission rate of 21% for microadenomas and 16% for macroadenomas was reported (31). Higher remission rates were seen in studies in which cabergoline was used, a longer duration of the treatment, and when shrinkage of the adenoma was >50%. The highest probability of remission can be expected when PRL serum levels are normal for a longer period of time and no visible tumor can be seen on MRI for at least 2 years. In general, the remission rates are low, especially in macroprolactinomas. When discontinuation is not feasible, a reduction in the dopamine agonist dose may well be possible without losing biochemical and symptom control.

Adverse Effects

Common side effects of dopamine agonist drugs are orthostatic hypotension, nausea, abdominal discomfort, and mental disturbances. Initiating a dopamine agonist in a low dose and a slow increase of dose may minimize gastrointestinal complaints and orthostatic hypotension. In general, cabergoline should be initiated 0.25 mg once or twice a week and ingested with some food and just before bedtime. Nausea is more common during bromocriptine use. Initial bromocriptine dose is twice daily 1.25 mg. In general, lower doses are accompanied with less severe side effects. However, some patients seem to be completely intolerant to dopamine agonists. For women, intravaginal administration of bromocriptine is reported to decrease the incidence of nausea (32).

Less frequent side effects are Raynaud's phenomenon, depression, alcohol intolerance, addictive behavior, and constipation.

Macroprolactinomas often infiltrated the base of the skull, when treated with dopamine agonist, CSF leakage as rhinorrhea may occur in case of a rapid tumor shrinkage (33). Early recognition of this complication is important due to a potential risk of meningitis. Withdrawal or tempering of the dopamine agonist dose is necessary when CSF leakage occurs and, if necessary or persistent, neurosurgical intervention.

Valvular Heart Disease

Ergot derivatives, such as cabergoline and pergolide, when given in high doses are associated with valvular heart disease in, for example, Parkinson's patients (27). This association appears to depend on dose and time of exposure. In Parkinson's disease, however, doses greatly exceed dose regimens as used in endocrine diseases.

Initial reports on cardiac valvulopathy in Parkinson's patients during cabergoline use triggered a number of studies assessing valvulopathy with cardiac ultrasonography in patients using cabergoline for hyperprolactinemia (34). Only one single study observed a higher frequency of moderate tricuspid regurgitation than age- and gender-matched subjects. None of the other studies observed any valvular regurgitation during long-term cabergoline treatment (34). Prolactinoma patients in these studies used standard doses of cabergoline of 0.5 to 1.5 mg/weekly. When prolactinoma patients use higher doses over longer time, a potential increased risk of developing valvular disease might exist although this has not been reported to date.

Nowadays, it is advised that cardiac ultrasonography should be performed approximately every 2 years in patients that use cabergoline >2 mg weekly. Also, dose adaptation to the lowest dose of cabergoline that is necessary to lower prolactin to the normal range is desirable (23).

Pregnancy

Initiation of a dopamine agonist can lead to rapid recovery of fertility even before menses is completely restored. Therefore, female patients of fertile age should be aware that initiation of dopamine agonist treatment could result in a pregnancy after only a few doses. The use of dopamine agonists during pregnancy is generally not recommended (13). In a selected group of macroprolactinomas, continuation of dopamine agonists may be prudent. Tumor behavior, invasiveness of the adenoma, and the relationship to vital structures, such as the optic chiasm, all influence the decision to continue dopaminergic treatment or not. Some reports do suggest that macroprolactinomas may grow or re-expand during pregnancy after discontinuation of dopamine agonists (13). Lactotroph hyperplasia of the normal pituitary gland may displace the prolactinoma, and high estrogen may stimulate tumor growth. In general, however, microprolactinomas as well as macroprolactinomas within the sellar bounderies seldom cause symptomatic tumor growth (13). Bromocriptine is the drug of choice during pregnancy. In more than 6000 pregnancies, no harmful effects were observed. Cabergoline seems to be safe as well; however, the number of reported pregnancies is low. Quinagoline has by far the lowest number of reported pregnancy outcomes and a poor safety profile and is therefore not recommended (13).

TABLE 9.1

Level of Evidence of Statements[a]

Statement	Level of Evidence
Dynamic testing to evaluate hyperprolactinemia should not be applied.	1b
A single prolactin assessment for the diagnosis of hyperprolactinemia is enough.	1b
Other causes of hyperprolactinemia should be excluded.	1a
Asymptomatic hyperprolactinemia does not need any treatment.	4
Microprolactinoma that only have irregular menses can be treated with oral contraceptives or cabergoline.	4
Cessation or switch of medication causes hyperprolactinemia.[b]	2b
Symptomatic micro- and macroadenomas should be treated with dopamine agonist.	1c
Cabergoline is the drug of choice because it has the highest efficacy in normalizing prolactin and tumor shrinkage.	1c
Women with prolactinomas need to discontinue dopamine agonist as soon as they know that they are pregnant.	3b
During pregnancy, prolactin assessment in prolactinoma patients is redundant.	1b
If dopamine agonists are indicated during pregnancy, bromocriptine is the drug of choice.	3a

[a] Summary of Endocrine Society Clinical Practice Guideline (13).
[b] Antipsychotic drugs should not be discontinued or switched without consent of the treating psychiatrist.

TABLE 9.2

Grade of Strength for Recommendations

Recommendation	Grade Strength
Macro-prolactin assessment is not useful in symptomatic individuals.	A
Usually, a single prolactin assessment will diagnose hyperprolactinemia.	A
Other causes of hyperprolactinemia should be excluded when a hyperprolactinemia diagnosis is established.	A
Symptomatic micro- or macroprolactinoma should be treated with adopamine agonist.	A
Asymptomatic microprolactinoma do not need treatment.	C
In collaboration with an endocrinologist; formal visual field assessment followed by MRI without gadolinium in pregnant women with prolactinomas that experience severe headaches with or without visual field changes.	B

REFERENCES

1. Bern HA, Nicoll CS. The comparative endocrinology of prolactin. Recent Prog Horm Res. 1968; 24:681–720.
2. Bole-Feysot C, Goffin V, Edery M, Binart N, Kelly PA. Prolactin (PRL) and its receptor: Actions, signal transduction pathways and phenotypes observed in PRL receptor knockout mice. Endocr Rev. 1998; 19(3):225–68.
3. Horseman ND, Gregerson KA. Prolactin actions. J Mol Endocrinol. 2014; 52(1):R95–106.
4. Grattan DR, Kokay IC. Prolactin: A pleiotropic neuroendocrine hormone. J Neuroendocrinol. 2008; 20(6):752–63.
5. Freeman ME, Kanyicska B, Lerant A, Nagy G. Prolactin: Structure, function, and regulation of secretion. Physiol Rev. 2000; 80(4):1523–631.
6. Matalka KZ, Ali DA. Stress-induced versus preovulatory and pregnancy hormonal levels in modulating cytokine production following whole blood stimulation. Neuroimmunomodulation. 2005; 12(6):366–74.
7. Pi XJ, Grattan DR. Increased prolactin receptor immunoreactivity in the hypothalamus of lactating rats. J Neuroendocrinol. 1999; 11(9):693–705.
8. Ben-Jonathan N, LaPensee CR, LaPensee EW. What can we learn from rodents about prolactin in humans? Endocr Rev. 2008; 29(1):1–41.
9. Larsen CM, Grattan DR. Prolactin, neurogenesis, and maternal behaviors. Brain Behav Immun. 2012; 26(2):201–9.
10. Chong BW, Kucharczyk W, Singer W, George S. Pituitary gland MR: A comparative study of healthy volunteers and patients with microadenomas. AJNR Am J Neuroradiol. 1994; 15(4):675–9.
11. Hall WA, Luciano MG, Doppman JL, Patronas NJ, Oldfield EH. Pituitary magnetic resonance imaging in normal human volunteers: Occult adenomas in the general population. Ann Intern Med. 1994; 120(10):817–20.
12. Kleinberg DL, Noel GL, Frantz AG. Galactorrhea: A study of 235 cases, including 48 with pituitary tumors. New Engl J Med. 1977; 296(11):589–600.
13. Melmed S, Casanueva FF, Hoffman AR, Kleinberg DL, Montori VM, Schlechte JA et al. Diagnosis and treatment of hyperprolactinemia: An Endocrine Society clinical practice guideline. J Clin Endocr Metab. 2011; 96(2):273–88.
14. Barkan AL, Chandler WF. Giant pituitary prolactinoma with falsely low serum prolactin: The pitfall of the "high-dose hook effect": Case report. Neurosurgery. 1998; 42(4):913–5; discussion 5–6.
15. Schlechte J, Dolan K, Sherman B, Chapler F, Luciano A. The natural history of untreated hyperprolactinemia: A prospective analysis. J Clin Endocrin Metab. 1989; 68(2):412–8.
16. Sluijmer AV, Lappohn RE. Clinical history and outcome of 59 patients with idiopathic hyperprolactinemia. Fertil Steril. 1992; 58(1):72–7.
17. Maiter D, Primeau V. 2012 update in the treatment of prolactinomas. Annal Endocrinol (Paris). 2012; 73(2):90–8.
18. Verhelst J, Abs R, Maiter D, van den Bruel A, Vandeweghe M, Velkeniers B et al. Cabergoline in the treatment of hyperprolactinemia: A study in 455 patients. J Clin Endocrinol Metab. 1999; 84(7):2518–22.
19. Schlechte J, Sherman B, Halmi N, VanGilder J, Chapler F, Dolan K et al. Prolactin-secreting pituitary tumors in amenorrheic women: A comprehensive study. Endocr Rev. 1980; 1(3):295–308.
20. Gillam MP, Molitch ME, Lombardi G, Colao A. Advances in the treatment of prolactinomas. Endocr Rev. 2006; 27(5):485–534.
21. Molitch ME. Pharmacologic resistance in prolactinoma patients. Pituitary. 2005; 8(1):43–52.
22. Molitch ME, Elton RL, Blackwell RE, Caldwell B, Chang RJ, Jaffe R et al. Bromocriptine as primary therapy for prolactin-secreting macroadenomas: Results of a prospective multicenter study. J Clin Endocrinol Metab. 1985; 60(4):698–705.
23. Neggers SJ, van der Lely AJ. Medical approach to pituitary tumors. Handb Clin Neurol. 2014; 124:303–16.
24. Vance ML, Evans WS, Thorner MO. Drugs five years later. Bromocriptine. Ann Intern Med. 1984; 100(1):78–91.
25. Biller BM, Molitch ME, Vance ML, Cannistraro KB, Davis KR, Simons JA et al. Treatment of prolactin-secreting macroadenomas with the once-weekly dopamine agonist cabergoline. J Clin Endocrinol Metab. 1996; 81(6):2338–43.

26. Kleinberg DL, Boyd AE, 3rd, Wardlaw S, Frantz AG, George A, Bryan N et al. Pergolide for the treatment of pituitary tumors secreting prolactin or growth hormone. New Engl J Med. 1983; 309(12):704–9.

27. Zanettini R, Antonini A, Gatto G, Gentile R, Tesei S, Pezzoli G. Valvular heart disease and the use of dopamine agonists for Parkinson's disease. New Engl J Med. 2007; 356(1):39–46.

28. van der Lely AJ, Brownell J, Lamberts SW. The efficacy and tolerability of CV 205-502 (a nonergot dopaminergic drug) in macroprolactinoma patients and in prolactinoma patients intolerant to bromocriptine. J Clin Endocrinol Metab. 1991; 72(5):1136–41.

29. Barlier A, Jaquet P. Quinagolide—A valuable treatment option for hyperprolactinaemia. Eur J Endocrinol. 2006; 154(2):187–95.

30. Ono M, Miki N, Kawamata T, Makino R, Amano K, Seki T et al. Prospective study of high-dose cabergoline treatment of prolactinomas in 150 patients. J Clin Endocrinol Metab. 2008; 93(12):4721–7.

31. Dekkers OM, Lagro J, Burman P, Jorgensen JO, Romijn JA, Pereira AM. Recurrence of hyperprolactinemia after withdrawal of dopamine agonists: Systematic review and meta-analysis. J Clin Endocrinol Metab. 2010; 95(1):43–51.

32. Kletzky OA, Vermesh M. Effectiveness of vaginal bromocriptine in treating women with hyperprolactinemia. Fertil Steril. 1989; 51(2):269–72.

33. Leong KS, Foy PM, Swift AC, Atkin SL, Hadden DR, MacFarlane IA. CSF rhinorrhoea following treatment with dopamine agonists for massive invasive prolactinomas. Clin Endocrinol (Oxf). 2000; 52(1):43–9.

34. Valassi E, Klibanski A, Biller BM. Clinical Review#: Potential cardiac valve effects of dopamine agonists in hyperprolactinemia. J Clin Endocrinol Metab. 2010; 95(3):1025–33.

10

Genetics of Anovulation*

Joop S. E. Laven

WHO 1 Anovulation

Hypogonadotrophic hypogonadism (HH) might result from combined pituitary hormonal deficiencies (CPHD) or from isolated gonadotropin-releasing hormone (Gn-RH), follicle-stimulating hormone (FSH), or luteinizing hormone (LH) deficiencies. For an extensive review, see Larson, Nokoff, and Meeks (1).

Among 195 individuals with combined pituitary hormonal deficiency, 13% were found to have mutations in one of five genes sequenced (*POU1F1, PROP1, LHX3, LHX4,* and *HESX1*). The yield was much higher for familial cases at 52%. Estimates of the prevalence of mutations in *PROP1* among patients with CPHD vary widely based on geography (due to founder effects) and presence or absence of family history. Turkish patients with CPHD had sequencing of *PROP1, POU1F1, LHX3,* and *HESX1* with mutations identified in 31% of patients. *PROP1* encodes a transcription factor critical for development of most lineages of anterior pituitary cells. *POU1F1* (formerly *PIT1*) is a transcription factor expressed in the subset of anterior pituitary cells that will secrete GH, TSH, and prolactin. Biallelic mutations in the gene cause deficiencies in these hormones. *HESX1* mutations are discussed below in conjunction with septo optic dysplasia (1).

LHX3 and *LHX4* mutations are rare causes of CPHD. The genes encode transcription factors critical for developing Rathke's pouch. Heterozygous mutations in *LHX4* can cause CPHD with a structurally abnormal pituitary gland, sella turcica, and cerebellum in some cases. A wide range of phenotypes have been noted, including individuals with only subtle subclinical hormone deficiencies. Biallelic mutations in *LHX3* result in CPHD with abnormal pituitary imaging and cervical spine anomalies. A syndrome of CPHD and hearing loss has also been described (1).

Sequence variants, deletions, and duplications of *SOX3*, a transcription factor, are associated with CPHD, pituitary imaging abnormalities, and other CNS morphological anomalies. *SOX3* is on the X chromosome, and manifestations are largely seen in males. A family with isolated GH deficiency in conjunction with intellectual disability due to *SOX3* mutation has been reported (1).

Deficiency of LH and FSH or HH, usually results from deficient action of hypothalamic Gn-RH. The association of anosmia with HH is known as Kallmann syndrome (KS). Abnormal development of the olfactory bulb impairs migration of the embryonic precursors of GnRH-secreting cells to the hypothalamus, resulting in the common association between anosmia and HH (2). There is a continuous spectrum of olfactory phenotypes among individuals with HH, and thus, we will often refer to HH/KS as a group rather than separately (1).

The first gene linked with KS, *KAL1*, resides on the X chromosome and encodes a secreted extracellular glycoprotein necessary for olfactory neuron axonal pathfinding (3). Fibroblast growth factor and prokineticin signaling are critical for olfactory bulb development and GnRH-secreting cell migration. Mutations in *FGFR1, FGF8, PROK2,* and *PROKR2* disrupt those signaling mechanisms and have been

---

* In this chapter no Levels of Evidence are provided because most of the data provided have not been derived from trials.

identified in patients with HH/KS (4–6). Compared to other etiologies of HH/KS, patients with KAL1 mutations are more likely to have very small testicular volume, complete absence of puberty, renal anomalies, and bimanual synkinesia (mirroring of the movements of one hand with the other). Patients with FGF8 and FGFR1 mutations are more likely to have cleft palate, dental anomalies, and syndactyly (1).

CHARGE syndrome is an acronym conveying the association of ocular coloboma, congenital heart defects, choanal atresia, growth restriction, intellectual disability, genital abnormalities, and ear abnormalities. Heterozygous mutations in the gene CHD7 cause CHARGE (7). The protein encoded by CHD7 is a chromatin modifier that regulates gene transcription and is expressed in the developing pituitary as well as other tissues. HH/KS represents the milder end of the phenotypic spectrum resulting from CHD7 mutations in comparison to the more severe CHARGE phenotype (8). Compared to patients with other gene mutations causing HH/KS, those with CHD7 mutations are more likely to have hearing loss (1).

Along with the aforementioned genes that are critical during embryogenesis of the olfactory bulb and hypothalamus, biallelic mutations within the genes encoding Gn-RH itself (GNRH1) and the Gn-RH receptor (GNRHR) can cause HH (9,10). Kisspeptin signaling is necessary for normal hypothalamic Gn-RH release and biallelic mutations in the gene encoding kisspeptin (KISS1) and the kisspeptin receptor (KISS1R) also result in HH (11,12). An additional signaling mechanism is now known to be necessary for normal Gn-RH release with mutations in the genes encoding neurokinin B (also known as tachykinin 3) and its receptor (TAC3 and TACR3) identified in families with recessively inherited HH/KS (1).

Complicating genetic counseling for HH/KS is the identification of patients with complex inheritance patterns. Digenic inheritance has been described in multiple families. Also, HH/KS appears to be a partially sex-limited phenotype: males with HH/KS outnumber females by a factor of about four. A small portion of the male predominance in HH/KS stems from the X-linked inheritance of KAL1 mutations. The fact that males may have physical exam findings apparent at birth (micropenis and undescended testes) could account for some ascertainment bias, but that alone also cannot account for such a wide disparity (1).

In HH/KS, the estimated prevalence of mutations in each gene depends on the specific phenotype in question. Generally speaking, genes with the highest prevalence of mutations are *FGFR1*, *KAL1*, *PROKR2*, *GNRHR*, and *CHD7* (13). None of these genes account for more than 10% of cases, and therefore, HH/KS is a phenotype usually more appropriate for panel testing rather than individual gene testing. In addition to those noted above, mutations in the genes encoding FEZF1, NR0B1, NSMF, WDR11, SEMA3A, HS6ST, SOX10, FGF17, IL17RD, SPRY4, DUSP6, and FLRT3 constitute rare causes of HH/KS. In the cases of some genes, it is not apparent whether mutations are sufficient to cause HH/KS in the absence of a second affected gene (1).

WHO 2 and PCOS

Because PCOS clusters within families, the syndrome is at least partially genetically determined. Earlier studies of the genetics of PCOS suggested an autosomal dominant mode of inheritance, but the recruitment of large families with multiple affected women likely biased these studies. Nowadays, PCOS is generally looked upon as being a complex polygenic disease that may involve the subtle interaction of environmental factors, susceptibility, and protective genomic variants (14).

The evidence for a common genetic background is derived from numerous studies either family or population based, candidate gene studies, and more recently, from genome-wide association studies (GWAS).

Two studies assessed the heritability of PCOS in twins by comparing the degree of concordance between mono- and dizygotic twin pairs. Both studies indicated that at least 50%–70% of the syndrome is attributable to genetic factors. Moreover, both studies showed that there is also evidence that these genetic factors do interact with unique environmental factors. Finally, they also showed that phenomena generally associated with the syndrome, that is, BMI, insulin resistance, and androgen levels, are genetically determined (15,16).

Evidence for the role of genetics in PCOS includes a well-documented familial clustering of PCOS with sisters more likely to be affected with signs and symptoms of the disorder, and first-degree relatives having higher rates of metabolic abnormalities including insulin resistance, decreased beta cell function, dyslipidemia, and MetS (17). Female as well as male siblings do exhibit higher levels of androgens. Moreover, the incidence of PCOS and PCOS characteristics is increased in sisters of affected probands within families (18,19).

Population-based studies have tested a large number of functional candidate genes for association or linkage with PCOS phenotypes, mostly ending with negative findings. However, a lack of universally accepted diagnostic criteria makes comparison of such studies problematic. A further problem is that the candidate gene approach relies upon some prior understanding of pathogenesis to determine the candidacy of the gene chosen with more than 20,000 genes to choose from within the human genome. Moreover, controversies and lack of consensus about how to define the syndrome hamper genetic research in this area. Finally, although more than 200 candidate genes have been studied up till now, the small sample size of most studies renders them underpowered, resulting in inconsistent results that, in most instances, have not been replicated in different independent samples (14). Genes or genetic variants that have been identified and replicated to a certain extent are FSH-R, TGF-β family members, insulin receptor and insulin signaling, WNT signaling (transcription factor 7 like 2 [TCG7L2]), fat and obesity-associated gene (FTO), and genetic variants in sex hormone binding globulin (SHBG) (20).

Thankfully, this limitation is overcome through use of the GWAS, the first of which in PCOS has already been published. The GWAS does not rely upon any a priori understanding of pathogenesis and, as such, holds the potential to reveal hitherto unexpected or even unknown pathogenic pathways that may be implicated in the development of PCOS (14). Recent genome-wide association studies in Han Chinese women with PCOS demonstrate 11 genetic loci that are associated with PCOS. The variants identified are in regions that contain genes important for gonadotropin action, genes that are associated with risk for type 2 diabetes, and other genes in which the relationship to PCOS is not yet clear. Replication studies have demonstrated that variants at several of these loci also confer risk for PCOS in women of European ethnicity (21,22). The strongest loci in Europeans contain genes for DENND1A and THADA with additional associations in loci containing the LHCGR and FSHR, YAP1, and RAB5/SUOX. The next steps in uncovering the pathophysiology borne out by these loci and variants will include mapping to determine the causal variant and gene, phenotype studies to determine whether these regions are associated with particular features of PCOS, and functional studies of the causal variant to determine the direct cause of PCOS based on the underlying genetics. The next years will be very exciting times as groups from around the world come together to further elucidate the genetic origins of PCOS (23). Recently, the functional roles of strong PCOS candidate loci focusing on FSHR, LHCGR, INSR, and DENND1A have been explored. Particularly, DENND1A seems a promising candidate because it is overexpressed in theca cells of PCOS patients. Moreover, forced overexpression in normal theca cells induced a PCOS-like phenotype in these cells whereas a knock-down of DENND1 in PCOS theca cells reduced androgen biosynthesis. It has been proposed that these candidates comprise a hierarchical signaling network by which DENND1A and probably LHCGR, INSR, RAB5B, adapter proteins, and associated downstream signaling cascades converge to regulate theca cell androgen biosynthesis. According to these authors future elucidation of these functional gene networks identified by future PCOS GWAS's will result in new diagnostic and therapeutic approaches for women with PCOS (24,25).

Several studies have examined candidate genes known to be involved in drug response and tried to identify predictive alleles. Such studies have identified genetic regions associated with a response to metformin, including a SNP in the serine-threonine kinase 11 gene associated with ovulation (26), and one in the OCT-1 transporter gene associated with a favorable reduction in cholesterol (27). Studies have associated FSHR gene polymorphisms with varying responses to gonadotropin ovulation induction, which may prove useful in treating women with PCOS (28,29).

WHO 3 or POI

Primary ovarian insufficiency is a condition that represents impaired ovarian function on a continuum with intermittent ovulation. This condition commonly leads to premature menopause, defined as cessation of ovulation prior to the age of 40 years. Potential etiologies for POI can be divided into genetic, autoimmune, and iatrogenic categories. Unfortunately, for most patients presenting with POI, the cause will remain unexplained (30).

Disorders that involve the X chromosome and loci that regulate germ cell development and viability are linked to POI. Turner syndrome (45,X) is associated with streak gonads and other stigmata, including short stature, a broad and webbed neck, coarctation of the aorta, a shortened fourth metacarpal, pigmented nevi, an ogival palate, cognitive deficits, vertebral abnormalities, and renal anomalies. The prevalence is about one in 2500 female births with 80% of cases being maternal in origin. A small percentage (up to 20%) of adolescents with Turner syndrome will menstruate spontaneously and exhibit breast development. In these cases, 45,X/46,XX mosaicism should be suspected (31).

Normal division of the centromere occurs in the longitudinal plane. When the centromere splits abnormally in the transverse plane, the resulting chromosome pair contains structurally identical arms with identical genes. Such isochromosomes of the X chromosome are also associated with POI. Isochromosomes for the long arm (q) of the X chromosome are the most common abnormality. These patients have streak gonads and tend to have the Turner stigmata. Genes of interest are ubiquitin-specific protease (USP9X) required for oogenesis and eye development, Zinc Finger (XZFX) associated with diminished germ cell numbers, bone morphogenic protein (BMP15) expressed in gonads and involved in folliculogenesis and short stature homeobox (SHOX) associated with short stature (31).

Similarly, microdeletions on the X chromosome are also detectable in women with POI. Gene mutations associated on the long arm of the X chromosome that are associated with POI are Xq13, XIST involved in X inactivation, Xq21–24, DIAPH2 (diaphanous), which aids in establishing cell polarity, reorganizing actin cytoskeleton, Xq21, POF1B, homozygotes individuals are affected whereas heterozygotes are unaffected, Xq25, XPNPEP2 and Xq22–23, ATZ receptor (angiotensin II type 2) expressed in fetal tissue and granulosa cells. The most commonly known mutations, FMR1 fragile X syndrome caused by an increased number of DNA base sequence CGG triplet repeats, lead to ineffective gene suppression, allowing other genes to become overly expressed. Fragile X syndrome is an inherited X-linked dominant disorder that is a leading cause of inherited cognitive disability. The FMR1 gene contains a CGG repeat present in the 5′-untranslated region, which can be unstable upon transmission to the next generation. The repeat is up to 55 CGGs long in the normal population. In patients with fragile X syndrome (FXS), a repeat length exceeding 200 CGGs (full mutation: FM) generally leads to methylation of the repeat and the promoter region, which is accompanied by silencing of the FMR1 gene. The absence of FMR1 protein, FMRP, seen in FM is the cause of the mental retardation in patients with FXS. The premutation (PM) is defined as 55-200 CGGs. Female PM carriers are at risk of developing primary ovarian insufficiency (32). Although there are regions on the short (p) and long arms (q) of the X chromosome that are designated ovarian genes (*POF1* and *POF2*, respectively), women with premature ovarian failure have been noted to have alterations outside these designated areas (31).

XX gonadal dysgenesis not associated with phenotypic anomalies are most commonly inherited in an autosomal recessive fashion. There is variance in phenotypic penetration noted among siblings (31). It has been challenging to identify the specific autosomal genes responsible for various forms of XX gonadal dysgenesis. There are sporadic cases associated with reciprocal autosomal translocations that have not been easily reproduced. Transgenic mouse models have been instrumental in the discovery of novel genetic determinants of gonadal development and failure and have informed researchers about possible mutations in women with POI. Genes identified to be associated with POI are 4p11–q12 (tyrosine kinase receptor), 12q22 (mast cell growth factor), 9q33 (nuclear receptor factor), 6p21.3 (DNA mismatch repair), and 18q21.3 (cell death repressor protein) (33).

Women who have phenotypic abnormalities in addition to ovarian insufficiency are likely to have the syndromic, as opposed to nonsyndromic (pathology confined to ovarian insufficiency), type of POI. These syndromes can be due to chromosomal abnormalities, such as Turner syndrome (monosomy X), or due to single gene mutations as is the case with galactosemia (*GALT*), pseudohypoparathyroidism type 1a (guanine nucleotide binding protein, α stimulating; *GNAS1*), progressive external ophthalmoplegia (polymerase [DNA directed], gamma; *POLG*), autoimmune polyglandular syndrome type 1 (autoimmune regulator; *AIRE*), ovarian leukodystrophy (eukaryotic translation initiation factor 2B, subunit 2 β; *EIF2B2*), Ataxia Telangiectasia (*ATM*), Demirhan syndrome (bone morphogenetic protein receptor, type 1B; *BMPR1B*), and BPESI (*FOXL2*) among others. Women with nonsyndromic and idiopathic POI were evaluated for the presence of *EIF2B2* and *GALT* mutations; however, no significant associations were found. Mice lacking *Atm*, *Aire*, or *Bmprlb* also have ovarian dysfunction although mutations in these genes have not been evaluated in patients with nonsyndromic and idiopathic POI. A SNP in *POLG* (rs2307449) associates with age at menopause (34).

Again numerous genetic variants have been investigated in different populations using a candidate gene approach. Most of the identified variants were associated with POI in one study whereas other studies failed to replicate these findings. For an extensive review see Wood and Rajkovic (34). Briefly, human FIGLA is expressed as early as 14 weeks of gestational age with a dramatic increase in transcripts by mid-gestation, suggesting a similarly conserved function of the human and mouse FIGLA proteins. Heterozygous mutations in FIGLA were found to be present in women with POI. Thus, haploinsufficiency of FIGLA likely causes accelerated loss of ovarian reserves in humans. NOBOX promotes primordial follicle activation. Human NOBOX expression within the ovary is oocyte specific, and observed from the primordial follicle to the metaphase II (MII) oocyte. NOBOX mutations were identified in a population of Caucasian women with POI. Forkhead box O3 (FOXO3), a transcription factor, is an important oocyte-specific regulator of primordial follicle activation and mutations in *FOXO3* were identified in women with POI. GDF9 and bone morphogenic protein 15 (BMP15) are oocyte-secreted growth factors that affect granulosa cell differentiation function. Three missense mutations in GDF9 were found in POI patients of Chinese or Indian descent. Two additional mutations were present in Caucasian women with POI. However, none of these variants were identified in Japanese women with POI. Forkhead box L2 (Foxl2), a transcriptional regulator, can repress primordial follicle activation through upregulation of AMH. FOXL2 activates the expression of AMH in granulosa cells of developing follicles, which, when secreted, can act in a paracrine manner to repress primordial follicle activation. Mutations in FOXL2 cause blepharophimosis–ptosis–epicanthus inversus syndrome, type I (BPESI) and II. Type I can present with POI. Multiple mutations in FOXL2 have also been found in women with nonsyndromic POI suggesting that mutations in FOXL2 may be a cause of idiopathic POI. Single nucleotide polymorphisms in genes of the estrogen receptor (ESR1), inhibin A (INHA) the FSH receptor (FSHR) and aromatase (CYP19A1) did produce conflicting results amongst different ethnic populations (34).

The genetic etiology of early menopause (EM) is largely unknown in the majority of cases. Recently, a GWAS, a meta-analysis of several genome-wide association studies, in 3493 women with EM and 13,598 controls from 10 independent studies has been performed. No novel genetic variants were discovered, but the 17 variants previously associated with normal age at natural menopause as a quantitative trait were also associated with EM as well as with POI. Thus, POI and early menopause do substantially overlap with normal menopause and is at least partly explained by the additive effects of the same polygenic variants. The combined effect of the common variants captured by the single nucleotide polymorphism arrays was estimated to account for approximately 30% of the variance in early menopause. Moreover, the distribution of risk alleles was similar in POI and early menopause individuals. The association between the combined 17 variants and the risk of early menopause was greater than the best validated non-genetic risk factor being smoking. Genetic markers of ovarian aging are present throughout life and thus may be superior to current best predictors, for example, AMH, inhibin B, and FSH levels, which are only reliable indicators toward the end of a woman's reproductive period which precedes actual menopause. As more genetic components of this trait are discovered, we will be able to include additional genetic data in predictive models for menopause age, giving women information about potential reproductive lifespan and enabling them to make informed reproductive choices (30).

REFERENCES

1. Larson A, Nokoff NJ, Meeks NJ. Genetic causes of pituitary hormone deficiencies. Discov Med. 2015; 19(104):175–83.
2. Teixeira L, Guimiot F, Dode C, Fallet-Bianco C, Millar RP, Delezoide AL et al. Defective migration of neuroendocrine GnRH cells in human arrhinencephalic conditions. J Clin Invest. 2010; 120(10):3668–72.
3. Legouis R, Hardelin JP, Levilliers J, Claverie JM, Compain S, Wunderle V et al. The candidate gene for the X-linked Kallmann syndrome encodes a protein related to adhesion molecules. Cell. 1991; 67(2):423–35.

4. Dode C, Rondard P. PROK2/PROKR2 Signaling and Kallmann Syndrome. Front Endocrinol (Lausanne). 2013; 4:19.

5. Falardeau J, Chung WC, Beenken A, Raivio T, Plummer L, Sidis Y et al. Decreased FGF8 signaling causes deficiency of gonadotropin-releasing hormone in humans and mice. J Clin Invest. 2008; 118(8):2822–31.

6. Pitteloud N, Acierno JS, Jr., Meysing A, Eliseenkova AV, Ma J, Ibrahimi OA et al. Mutations in fibroblast growth factor receptor 1 cause both Kallmann syndrome and normosmic idiopathic hypogonadotropic hypogonadism. Proc Natl Acad Sci U S A. 2006; 103(16):6281–6.

7. Lalani SR, Hefner MA, Belmont JW, Davenport SLH. CHARGE Syndrome. In: Pagon RA, Adam MP, Ardinger HH, Wallace SE, Amemiya A, Bean LJH et al., editors. Gene Reviews (R). Seattle (WA) 1993.

8. Kim HG, Bhagavath B, Layman LC. Clinical manifestations of impaired GnRH neuron development and function. Neurosignals. 2008; 16(2–3):165–82.

9. Bouligand J, Ghervan C, Tello JA, Brailly-Tabard S, Salenave S, Chanson P et al. Isolated familial hypogonadotropic hypogonadism and a GNRH1 mutation. N Engl J Med. 2009; 360(26):2742–8.

10. de Roux N, Young J, Misrahi M, Genet R, Chanson P, Schaison G et al. A family with hypogonadotropic hypogonadism and mutations in the gonadotropin-releasing hormone receptor. N Engl J Med. 1997; 337(22):1597–602.

11. de Roux N, Genin E, Carel JC, Matsuda F, Chaussain JL, Milgrom E. Hypogonadotropic hypogonadism due to loss of function of the KiSS1-derived peptide receptor GPR54. Proc Natl Acad Sci U S A. 2003; 100(19):10972–6.

12. Topaloglu AK, Tello JA, Kotan LD, Ozbek MN, Yilmaz MB, Erdogan S et al. Inactivating KISS1 mutation and hypogonadotropic hypogonadism. N Engl J Med. 2012; 366(7):629–35.

13. Bianco SD, Kaiser UB. The genetic and molecular basis of idiopathic hypogonadotropic hypogonadism. Nat Rev Endocrinol. 2009; 5(10):569–76.

14. Barber TM, Franks S. Genetics of polycystic ovary syndrome. Front Horm Res. 2013; 40:28–39.

15. Jahanfar S, Eden JA, Warren P, Seppala M, Nguyen TV. A twin study of polycystic ovary syndrome. Fertil Steril. 1995; 63(3):478–86.

16. Vink JM, Sadrzadeh S, Lambalk CB, Boomsma DI. Heritability of polycystic ovary syndrome in a Dutch twin-family study. J Clin Endocrinol Metab. 2006; 91(6):2100–4.

17. Diamanti-Kandarakis E, Kandarakis H, Legro RS. The role of genes and environment in the etiology of PCOS. Endocrine. 2006; 30(1):19–26.

18. Sam S, Coviello AD, Sung YA, Legro RS, Dunaif A. Metabolic phenotype in the brothers of women with polycystic ovary syndrome. Diabetes Care. 2008; 31(6):1237–41.

19. Legro RS, Driscoll D, Strauss JF, 3rd, Fox J, Dunaif A. Evidence for a genetic basis for hyperandrogenemia in polycystic ovary syndrome. Proc Natl Acad Sci U S A. 1998; 95(25):14956–60.

20. Kosova G, Urbanek M. Genetics of the polycystic ovary syndrome. Mol Cell Endocrinol. 2013; 373(1–2):29–38.

21. Day FR, Hinds DA, Tung JY, Stolk L, Styrkarsdottir U, Saxena R, Bjonnes A et al. Causal mechanisms and balancing selection inferred from genetic associations with polycystic ovary syndrome. Nat Commun. 2015; 6:8464. doi:10.1038/ncomms9464.

22. Hayes MG, Urbanek M, Ehrmann DA, Armstrong LL, Lee JY, Sisk R, Karaderi T et al. Genome-wide association of polycystic ovary syndrome implicates alterations in gonadotropin secretion in European ancestry populations. Nat Commun. 2015; 6:7502. doi:10.1038/ncomms8502.

23. Welt CK, Duran JM. Genetics of polycystic ovary syndrome. Semin Reprod Med. 2014; 32(3):177–82.

24. McAllister JM, Legro RS, Modi BP, Strauss JF, 3rd. Functional genomics of PCOS: From GWAS to molecular mechanisms. Trends Endocrinol Metab. 2015; 26(3):118–24.

25. McAllister JM, Modi B, Miller BA, Biegler J, Bruggeman R, Legro RS et al. Overexpression of a DENND1A isoform produces a polycystic ovary syndrome theca phenotype. Proc Natl Acad Sci U S A. 2014; 111(15):E1519–27.

26. Legro RS, Barnhart HX, Schlaff WD, Carr BR, Diamond MP, Carson SA et al. Ovulatory response to treatment of polycystic ovary syndrome is associated with a polymorphism in the STK11 gene. J Clin Endocrinol Metab. 2008; 93(3):792–800.

27. Malavasi EL, Kelly V, Nath N, Gambineri A, Dakin RS, Pagotto U et al. Functional effects of poly-morphisms in the human gene encoding 11 beta-hydroxysteroid dehydrogenase type 1 (11 beta-HSD1): A sequence variant at the translation start of 11 beta-HSD1 alters enzyme levels. Endocrinology. 2010; 151(1):195–202.

28. Valkenburg O, van Santbrink EJ, Konig TE, Themmen AP, Uitterlinden AG, Fauser BC et al. Follicle-stimulating hormone receptor polymorphism affects the outcome of ovulation induction in normogo-nadotropic (World Health Organization class 2) anovulatory subfertility. Fertil Steril. 2015; 103(4):1081–8 e3.

29. Valkenburg O, Uitterlinden AG, Piersma D, Hofman A, Themmen AP, de Jong FH et al. Genetic poly-morphisms of GnRH and gonadotrophic hormone receptors affect the phenotype of polycystic ovary syndrome. Hum Reprod. 2009; 24(8):2014–22.

30. Perry JR, Corre T, Esko T, Chasman DI, Fischer K, Franceschini N et al. A genome-wide associa-tion study of early menopause and the combined impact of identified variants. Hum Mol Genet. 2013; 22(7):1465–72.

31. Cox L, Liu JH. Primary ovarian insufficiency: An update. Int J Womens Health. 2014; 6:235–43.

32. Willemsen R, Levenga J, Oostra BA. CGG repeat in the FMR1 gene: Size matters. Clin Genet. 2011; 80(3):214–25.

33. Simpson JL, Rajkovic A. Ovarian differentiation and gonadal failure. Am J Med Genet. 1999; 89(4):186–200.

34. Wood MA, Rajkovic A. Genomic markers of ovarian reserve. Semin Reprod Med. 2013; 31(6):399–415.

11

Diagnosis of Anovulation

Joop S. E. Laven

Introduction

Generally, anovulation is diagnosed based on the assessment of both gonadotrophins FSH and LH along with a measurement of serum estradiol levels. In case LH as well as FSH serum concentrations are low and estradiol levels are also in the lower limit of detection, a central defect should be suspected. Generally, such defect leads to a hypogonadotropic hypogonadism, which is classified according to the World Health Organization classification as WHO 1 anovulation (1). In case gonadotrophin levels are elevated and estradiol serum concentrations are low, a peripheral, that is, ovarian defect should be suspected. Typically in these women, FSH levels are higher compared to LH serum concentrations. This so-called monotropic rise is caused by a lack of inhibin feedback upon FSH secretion from the pituitary and is pathognomonic for ovarian failure. In general, these women are classified as suffering from hypergonadotropic hypogonadism and categorized into the WHO 3 class (1). Finally, in the majority of cases FSH and LH levels as well as estradiol concentrations are normal. These cases are generally referred to as having normogonadotropic normo-estrogenic anovulation, and they are categorized into the WHO 2 class (1). Depending on what definition is used, a smaller or greater number of these women can also be diagnosed as having polycystic ovary syndrome (PCOS) (2,3) (see Figure 11.1).

WHO 1 Hypogonadotropic Hypogonadism (HH)

Clinical presentation of HH depends on the time of onset (i.e., congenital vs. acquired), the severity of the defect, and the presence of associated conditions. Typically, the diagnosis of congenital HH is made during the second or third decade of life when the patients present with delayed pubertal onset (i.e., after the age of 14 years), absent or poorly developed secondary sexual characteristics, primary amenorrhea, eunuchoid proportions, or infertility. For an extensive review, see Silveira and Latronico (4). Newborn girls have no obvious abnormal findings that might provide clues to the diagnosis. Most commonly, the diagnosis cannot be made until the expected time of puberty onset except in the neonatal period when gonadotropin and sexual steroid levels are expected to be elevated. The presence of anosmia is suggestive of Kallmann syndrome, and if the child is too young to undergo olfaction tests, a magnetic resonance imaging (MRI) scan showing absent or abnormal olfactory bulbs or sulci strongly suggests the diagnosis. Nevertheless, it is important to note that a normal MRI does not rule out the disease because normal olfactory bulbs can be present in up to one in five Kallmann syndrome patients. Adult-onset HH is characterized in women by secondary amenorrhea, decreased libido, infertility, and osteoporosis (4).

The evidence of hypogonadotropic hypogonadistic status in women indicates the diagnosis of HH. Rarely, selective deficiency of LH or FSH can occur due to inactivating mutations of the specific

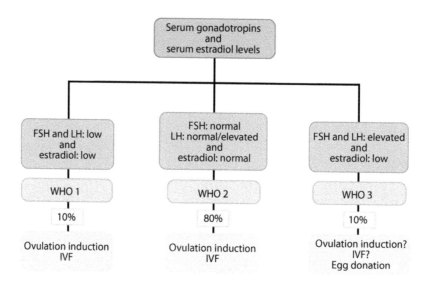

FIGURE 11.1   The initial assessment of the anovulatory patient.

β-subunits (5,6). Anterior pituitary function must be investigated to rule out a more complex endocrine disorder with multiple hormone deficiencies (4).

Although widely used, the practical value of the Gn-RH test has been questionable because of its low cost-effectiveness. Indeed, the Gn-RH test provides no extra diagnostic information relative to baseline gonadotropin levels, and in HH patients, the response to the Gn-RH test is highly variable. Thyroid function should be screened by measuring serum TSH levels. IGF-I can be used to evaluate the somatotropic axis. To assess the pituitary adrenal axis, morning cortisol should be measured. Stimulatory tests should be reserved for situations in which the basal hormone measurements are not helpful or if there is strong clinical evidence of a multiple pituitary hormone deficiency (4).

Anosmia can be easily diagnosed by questioning the patient whereas olfactometry, such as the University of Pennsylvania Smell Identification Test, is necessary to determine reliably whether olfaction is normal or partially defective (7). Indeed, IHH patients display a broad spectrum of olfactory function with a significant hyposmic phenotype. Accurate olfactory phenotyping in IHH subjects can inform the pathophysiology of this condition and guide genetic testing (7).

MRI of the hypothalamo-pituitary region is very useful in the management of HH. MRI can demonstrate a malformation, an expansive or infiltrative disorder of the hypothalamo-pituitary region. However, the cost-effectiveness of an MRI scan to exclude pituitary and/or hypothalamic tumors is unknown according to the recent clinical practice guideline (4,8). Pituitary and/or hypothalamic tumors should be investigated using MRI in patients with multiple pituitary hormone deficiency, persistent hyperprolactinemia, or symptoms of tumor mass effect (headache, visual impairment, or visual field defect) or secondary amenorrhea. In the presence of suspected functional causes of HH, such as severe obesity, nutritional disorders, and drugs, MRI is not indicated. Additionally, MRI with specific cuts for evaluating the olfactory tract can be helpful in the diagnosis of Kallmann syndrome. Evidence of unilateral or bilateral hypoplastic agenesis olfactory bulbs and hypoplastic anterior pituitary is pathognomonic of Kallmann syndrome (4).

Renal ultrasound examination is usually recommended to patients with syndromic IHH, such as Kallmann syndrome, independent of the genetic basis although it is well known that unilateral kidney agenesis may be more prevalent in patients with KAL1 defects. The genetic assessment is usually the last step in the congenital IHH investigation, and complete clinical characterization could certainly help in the gene selection. Bone mineral density of the lumbar spine, femoral neck, and hip is recommended at the initial diagnosis of HH and after 1 to 2 years of sex steroid therapy in hypogonadal patients with osteoporosis or low trauma fracture (4).

In a minority of cases and mainly in familial forms, genetic autosomal causes have been found. These cases are related to mutations of genes impinging the functioning of the pituitary–hypothalamic pathways involved in the normal secretion of LH and FSH (mutations of GnRHR, GnRH1, KISS1R/GPR54, TAC3, TACR3), which are always associated to isolated non-syndromic congenital HH without anosmia. Some cases of mutations of FGFR1 and, more rarely, of its ligand FGF8 or of PROKR2 or its ligand PROK2 have been shown in women suffering from Kallmann syndrome or its hyposmic or normosmic variant. In complex syndromic causes (mutations of CHD7, leptin and leptin receptor anomalies, Prader-Willi syndrome, etc.), diagnosis of the CHH cause is most often suspected or set down before the age of puberty by reason of the associated clinical signs, but some rare cases of paucisymptomatic syndromic causes can initially be revealed during adolescence, such as isolated non-syndromic CHH or Kallmann syndrome (8).

WHO 2 Normogonadotropic Normo-Estrogenic Anovulation

Most anovulatory patients (approximately 80%) present with serum FSH and estradiol levels within the normal range. Hence, they are classified as being WHO class 2 patients. Polycystic ovary syndrome (PCOS) is a common but poorly defined heterogeneous clinical entity. Historically, characteristic ovarian abnormalities represented a hallmark of the syndrome. Because several etiological factors may lead to a similar end point (i.e., polycystic ovaries), the development of a clinically applicable classification of the syndrome has proven difficult. Clinical, morphological, biochemical, endocrine, and molecular studies have identified an array of underlying abnormalities and added to the confusion concerning the pathophysiology of the disease (3). Nowadays, there is consensus that for clinical purposes PCOS should be diagnosed according the to the Rotterdam consensus (2,9) (see Figure 11.2).

According to the Rotterdam consensus, the diagnosis of PCOS should be made if two of the three following criteria are met: androgen excess, ovulatory dysfunction, or polycystic ovarian morphology (PCOM) (9).

Anovulation may manifest as frequent bleeding at intervals <21 days or infrequent bleeding at intervals of >35 days (2). Occasionally, bleeding may be anovulatory despite falling at a normal interval (25–35 days). A mid-luteal progesterone documenting anovulation may help with the diagnosis if bleeding intervals appear to suggest regular ovulation (10).

Clinical hyperandrogenism may include hirsutism, that is, excessive terminal hair that appears in a male pattern, acne, or androgenic alopecia. Generally hirsutism might be assessed using the Ferriman-Gallwey score. In the modified method, hair growth is rated from 0 (no growth of terminal hair) to 4 (extensive hair growth) in each of nine predefined locations. A patient's score may therefore range from a minimum score of 0 to a maximum score of 36. In Caucasian women, a score of 8 or higher is regarded as indicative of androgen excess. With other ethnic groups, the amount of hair expected for that ethnicity should be considered (9).

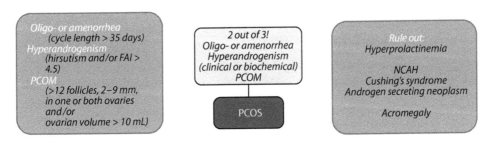

FIGURE 11.2 The Rotterdam consensus diagnostic criteria for PCOS.

Biochemical hyperandrogenism is defined as elevated serum androgen level and typically includes an elevated total, bioavailable, or free serum T level. Given variability in testosterone levels and the poor standardization of assays, it is difficult to define an absolute level that is diagnostic of PCOS or other causes of hyperandrogenism (9).

The PCO morphology has been defined by the presence of 12 or more follicles 2–9 mm in diameter and/or an ovarian volume exceeding 10 ml (without a cyst or dominant follicle) in either ovary (11). Critical analysis of the literature showed that ovarian volume had less diagnostic potential for PCOM compared with the follicle number per ovary. Moreover, if one is using more modern ultrasound machines with higher probe frequencies, the cutoff for PCOM should be probably higher, up to 25 or more per ovary (12).

Other disorders that might mimic the clinical features of PCOS are to be excluded. These include, in all women, thyroid disease, hyperprolactinemia, and non-classic congenital adrenal hyperplasia (primarily 21-hydroxylase deficiency). Hence patients with WHO 2 anovulation should screened for abnormal TSH serum levels, hyperprolactinemia as well as elevated levels of 17-hydroxy progesterone. Elevated levels of 17-OH-progesterone are only pathologic in combination with concomitant low values of progesterone as levels rise with ovulation. Signs of virilization, including change in voice, male pattern androgenic alopecia, and clitoromegaly or a rapid onset of hyperandrogenic associated symptoms should be evaluated for androgen producing tumors by assessing other androgens (i.e., Androstenedione, DHEA, and DHEAS) as well. Many of the signs and symptoms of PCOS can overlap with Cushing's, such as striae, obesity, and dorsocervical fat (i.e., buffalo hump, glucose intolerance). However, Cushing's is more likely to be present when a large number of signs and symptoms, especially those with high discriminatory index (e.g., myopathy, plethora, violaceous striae, easy bruising) are present, and this presentation should lead to screening using several available tests. A 24-hour urinary collection identifying an elevated level of free cortisol or a measurement of an elevated late night salivary cortisol might be used. An overnight dexamethasone suppression test showing a failure to suppress morning serum cortisol level the day after dexamethasone was given is also indicative for Cushing's disease. Finally, oligomenorrhea and skin changes (thickening, tags, hirsutism, hyperhidrosis) suggestive for acromegaly might as well overlap with PCOS. However, headaches, peripheral vision loss, enlarged jaw (macrognathia), frontal bossing, macroglossia, increased shoe and glove size, etc., are indications for screening for acromegaly. The latter should be done by assessing (elevated) free IGF-I serum levels eventually in combination with an MRI of the pituitary (9).

The diagnosis of PCOS in an adolescent girl might be made based on the presence of clinical and/ or biochemical evidence of hyperandrogenism (after exclusion of other pathologies) in the presence of persistent oligomenorrhea. Anovulatory symptoms and PCOM are not sufficient to make a diagnosis in adolescents as they may be evident in normal stages in reproductive maturation (13).

Although there are currently no diagnostic criteria for PCOS in peri-menopausal and postmenopausal women, we suggest that a presumptive diagnosis of PCOS can be based upon a well-documented long-term history of oligomenorrhea and hyperandrogenism during the reproductive years. The presence of PCOM on ultrasound would provide additional supportive evidence although this is less likely in a peri-menopausal woman (9).

WHO 3 Hypergonadotropic Hypogonadism (Premature Ovarian Insufficiency [POI])

In patients presenting with elevated gonadotrophins and, more specifically, a monotropic rise in FSH in combination with low levels of estradiol are to be diagnosed with premature ovarian insufficiency (POI).

This condition commonly leads to premature menopause, defined as cessation of ovulation prior to the age of 40 years. For a comprehensive review, see Cox and Liu (14).

The diagnosis should be confirmed by obtaining two consecutive FSH measurements revealing levels in the menopausal range (>40 IU/L) at least 1 month apart in the setting of 6 months of amenorrhea. Patients typically present with either primary or secondary oligomenorrhea or amenorrhea and may exhibit increasing symptoms of oestrogen deficiency. Patients may present with a shortening or increase in the inter-menstrual cycle interval or menstrual irregularities, including oligomenorrhea, dysfunctional uterine bleeding, or amenorrhea. Women may note symptoms of estrogen deficiency, such as vasomotor symptoms (i.e., hot flashes and night sweats), mood and sleeping disturbances, and atrophic vaginitis giving rise to dyspareunia although these later symptoms are usually delayed. Patients can also experience long-term consequences of hypo-estrogenism, which include osteoporosis, accelerated cardiovascular aging, and neurocognitive disorders. Infertility is another consequence of POI. Although most patients will present with amenorrhea, about 50% will have varying degrees of residual ovarian function. It is estimated that approximately 5%–10% are able to conceive spontaneously (14).

Unfortunately, standardized diagnostic criteria for POI have yet to be established. It is advisable to perform a complete history and physical examination to exclude secondary causes of amenorrhea. These conditions include pregnancy, polycystic ovarian syndrome, hypothalamic amenorrhea, chronic medical illness secondary to poorly controlled diabetes or celiac disease, lifestyle habits (extreme exercise, poor caloric intake), hypothalamic or pituitary lesions, hyperprolactinemia, hypothyroidism, and hyperthyroidism. The screening history should also focus on a family history of early menopause and previous ovarian/pelvic surgery as well as chemotherapy or radiation therapy, which may identify a cause. The clinician should probe for a personal or family history of autoimmune disorders (e.g., thyroid disorders, diabetes, Addison's disease, vitiligo, systemic lupus, rheumatoid arthritis, celiac disease), fragile X syndrome, or intellectual disability (15).

The physical examination should focus on body habitus and evidence of normal secondary sexual characteristics as well as evidence of vaginal atrophy secondary to hypo-estrogenism. For women with amenorrhea, apart from a determination of FSH, LH, and estradiol, laboratory testing should include human chorionic gonadotropin (hCG) to exclude pregnancy, TSH for thyroid disease screening, prolactin measurement, to exclude hyperpolactinemia. Additional testing should also include a peripheral karyotype (to look for Turner syndrome or 45,X/46,XX mosaicism or Xq isochromosome), a fragile X screen (especially in familiar cases), screening for antibodies against adrenal, thyroid tissue, and thyroid stimulating hormone receptors and ovarian tissue. Should a Y chromosome be identified, the patient should be counseled regarding gonadal removal because these individuals have an increased potential for malignancy (14).

Because some women with POI do have periodic estrogen production, administering a progesterone withdrawal test may not be particularly helpful. Transabdominal (in case of virginity) or transvaginal ultrasound might be helpful in assessing a low antral follicle count or even absent follicles in both ovaries. Findings of a normal ovarian size/volume and presence of a high antral ovarian follicle count (AFC) makes the diagnosis of POI less likely. For those women with diminished ovarian function, options to assess ovarian reserve include cycle day 3 FSH levels, anti-Müllerian hormone (AMH), inhibin B, and transvaginal ultrasound-determined AFC. Generally, a monotropic rise in FSH is pathognomonic for POI. To further substantiate the diagnosis, low or undetectable AMH as well as inhibin B levels might be helpful. Similarly, an AFC below 3 might be indicative for a substantially reduced ovarian reserve (16).

As a consequence of decreased estrogen levels, women with POI often do not achieve peak bone density and may experience loss of bone mass. If hormone therapy is initiated and the woman has not experienced fractures, it is not necessary to do bone mineral density testing (14).

TABLE 11.1

Level of Evidence of Statements

Statement	Level of Evidence
Hypogonadotropic hypogonadism is characterized by low levels of FSH and LH along with low levels of estradiol; it is classified as WHO class 1 anovulation.	2
In HH (WHO class 1) patients, anosmia or hyposmia is suggestive for Kallmann syndrome.	2
Normogonadotropic normo-estrogenic anovulation is characterized by normal levels of FSH, LH, and estradiol; it is classified as WHO class 2 anovulation. The majority of these women also suffer from polycystic ovary syndrome (PCOS).	2
PCOS should be diagnosed according to the Rotterdam consensus.	3
According to the Rotterdam consensus, the diagnosis of PCOS should be made if two of the three following criteria are met: androgen excess, ovulatory dysfunction, or polycystic ovarian morphology (PCOM).	2
A normal bleeding interval is between 21 and 35 days.	3
Hirsutism is defined as a Ferriman-Gallwey score of 8 or higher. Biochemical hyperandrogenism is defined as an elevated testosterone level or an elevated free androgen index (FAI) [T × 100/SHBG].	3
PCOM is defined as an increased number of follicles per ovary. The cutoff depends on the frequency of the transducer used. In case a FNPO is not assessable, ovarian volume might be used.	2
Cutoff values for clinical and biochemical hyperandrogenism are laboratory and age as well as ethnicity dependent.	2
Other causes of anovulation (thyroid disease or hyperpolactinemia) or HA (classical and non-classical forms of congenital adrenal hyperplasia, adrenal tumors, and Cushing's disease) should be ruled out before the diagnosis of PCOS can be made.	2
Hypergonadotropic hypogonadism is characterized by elevated levels of FSH and LH along with low levels of estradiol; it is classified as WHO class 3 anovulation. The monotropic rise in FSH is pathognomonic in these patients.	2
Patients with POI typically present with primary or secondary amenorrhea.	2
POI is often accompanied by complaints, such as hot flashes, night sweats, neurocognitive complaints as well as sexual problems such as loss of libido and dyspareunia.	2
Assessment of AMH levels or AFC measurements might aid the diagnosis of anovulatory infertility.	3

TABLE 11.2

Grade of Strength for Recommendations

Recommendation	Grade Strength
In anovulatory patients, FSH, LH, and estradiol should be determined during the initial workup. To rule out other pathologies, prolactin, TSH, and early morning cortisol should be measured too.	B
In anovulatory patients, a thorough history should be taken focusing on lifestyle habits (extreme exercise, poor caloric intake, and obesity), signs of other endocrinopathies (i.e., hypothalamic or pituitary lesions, hyperprolactinemia, hypothyroidism, and hyperthyroidism). The screening history should also focus on a family history of irregular cycles, HA, or early menopause along with a family history of autoimmune disorders (e.g., thyroid disorders, diabetes, Addison's disease, vitiligo, systemic lupus, rheumatoid arthritis, celiac disease), fragile X syndrome, or intellectual disability.	B
The physical examination should focus on body habitus, evidence of normal secondary sexual characteristics, hirsutism, and alopecia as well as evidence of vaginal atrophy secondary to hypo-estrogenism.	B
MRI might aid in the diagnosis of Kallmann syndrome and is mandatory in cases with multiple endocrinopathies to rule out tumors in the pituitary or midbrain regions.	B
Gn-RH testing is not cost-effective and not recommended. IGF-1 measurements are only recommended in WHO 1 patients without any sigs of pubertal development.	C
Accurate olfactory phenotyping in IHH subjects can inform the pathophysiology of this condition and guide genetic testing.	C
Renal ultrasound examination is recommended to patients with syndromic IHH, such as Kallmann syndrome, independent of the genetic basis.	C
Bone mineral density of the lumbar spine, femoral neck, and hip is recommended at the initial diagnosis of HH and after 1 to 2 years of sex steroid therapy in hypogonadal patients with osteoporosis or low trauma fracture.	C
PCOS should be diagnosed according to the Rotterdam consensus.	B
Clinical hyperandrogenism (HA) should be assessed using the Ferriman-Gallwey score. Biochemical HA should preferably be assessed according to the available assay (either LCM/S or RIA assays).	B
Adolescent PCOS is diagnosed if all three Rotterdam consensus characteristics of PCOS are present.	C
In postmenopausal women, the diagnosis is impossible to make but should be considered in women with a clear-cut history of irregular menstrual periods and signs of hyperandrogenism, such as hirsutism.	C
The diagnosis should be confirmed by obtaining two consecutive FSH measurements revealing levels in the menopausal range (>40 IU/L) at least 1 month apart in the setting of 6 months of amenorrhea.	B
Women with POI should be screened for X chromosome aberrations and for FMR1 gene (pre)mutations.	B
Women with POI should also be screened for auto-antibodies against adrenal, thyroid tissue, and thyroid stimulating hormone receptors and ovarian tissue.	B
Measurement of AMH or AFC is not routinely recommended for women with POI.	C
BMD measurements are not recommended in women with POI who have been treated with HRT since the time of diagnosis.	B

REFERENCES

1. Rabau E, Serr DM, Mashiach S, Insler V, Salomy M, Lunenfeld B. Current concepts in the treatment of anovulation. Br Med J. 1967; 4(5577):446–9.
2. Rotterdam EA-SPcwg. Revised 2003 consensus on diagnostic criteria and long-term health risks related to polycystic ovary syndrome (PCOS). Hum Reprod. 2004; 19(1):41–7.
3. Laven JS, Imani B, Eijkemans MJ, Fauser BC. New approach to polycystic ovary syndrome and other forms of anovulatory infertility. Obstet Gynecol Surv. 2002; 57(11):755–67.
4. Silveira LF, Latronico AC. Approach to the patient with hypogonadotropic hypogonadism. J Clin Endocrinol Metab. 2013; 98(5):1781–8.
5. Lofrano-Porto A, Barra GB, Giacomini LA, Nascimento PP, Latronico AC, Casulari LA et al. Luteinizing hormone beta mutation and hypogonadism in men and women. N Engl J Med. 2007; 357(9):897–904.
6. Layman LC. Genetics of human hypogonadotropic hypogonadism. Am J Med Genet. 1999; 89(4):240–8.

7. Lewkowitz-Shpuntoff HM, Hughes VA, Plummer L, Au MG, Doty RL, Seminara SB et al. Olfactory phenotypic spectrum in idiopathic hypogonadotropic hypogonadism: Pathophysiological and genetic implications. J Clin Endocrinol Metab. 2012; 97(1):E136–44.

8. Bry-Gauillard H, Trabado S, Bouligand J, Sarfati J, Francou B, Salenave S et al. Congenital hypogonadotropic hypogonadism in females: Clinical spectrum, evaluation and genetics. Ann Endocrinol (Paris). 2010; 71(3):158–62.

9. Legro RS, Arslanian SA, Ehrmann DA, Hoeger KM, Murad MH, Pasquali R et al. Diagnosis and treatment of polycystic ovary syndrome: An Endocrine Society clinical practice guideline. J Clin Endocrinol Metab. 2013; 98(12):4565–92.

10. Burgers JA, Fong SL, Louwers YV, Valkenburg O, de Jong FH, Fauser BC et al. Oligoovulatory and anovulatory cycles in women with polycystic ovary syndrome (PCOS): What's the difference? J Clin Endocrinol Metab. 2010; 95(12):E485–9.

11. Balen AH, Laven JS, Tan SL, Dewailly D. Ultrasound assessment of the polycystic ovary: International consensus definitions. Hum Reprod Update. 2003; 9(6):505–14.

12. Dewailly D, Lujan ME, Carmina E, Cedars MI, Laven J, Norman RJ et al. Definition and significance of polycystic ovarian morphology: A task force report from the Androgen Excess and Polycystic Ovary Syndrome Society. Hum Reprod Update. 2014; 20(3):334–52.

13. Witchel SF, Oberfield S, Rosenfield RL, Codner E, Bonny A, Ibanez L et al. The diagnosis of polycystic ovary syndrome during adolescence. Horm Res Paediatr. 2015.

14. Cox L, Liu JH. Primary ovarian insufficiency: An update. Int J Womens Health. 2014; 6:235–43.

15. Nelson LM. Clinical practice. Primary ovarian insufficiency. N Engl J Med. 2009; 360(6):606–14.

16. Rafique S, Sterling EW, Nelson LM. A new approach to primary ovarian insufficiency. Obstet Gynecol Clin North Am. 2012; 39(4):567–86.

12

Ovulation Induction versus Controlled Ovarian Hyperstimulation

Ben J. Cohlen

Introduction

Chronic anovulation is a common feature in infertile couples. It is unknown how many couples suffer from anovulation in the general population, but estimates vary between 5% and 15%. Being a sign rather than a disease, chronic anovulation is treated in various ways, depending on the underlying cause.

Although with ovulation induction, treatment is started to regain monthly mono-ovulation, the aim of treatment in controlled ovarian hyperstimulation is the development and ovulation of at least two dominant follicles to improve pregnancy chances in an ovulatory patient. However, two very different treatment strategies, ovulation induction (OI) and controlled ovarian hyperstimulation (COH), are often mixed up, which might result in unnecessary complications (Chapters 23 through 26).

In this chapter, both treatment modalities are defined and discussed.

Definitions

The WHO-ICMART committees defined ovulation induction as follows: pharmacologic treatment of women with anovulation or oligo-ovulation with the intention of inducing normal ovulatory cycles (1). From this definition, we can conclude that the intention of OI is the release of one oocyte per cycle, resembling normal ovulatory cycles. Thus, the goal of OI should be monthly mono-follicular development and mono-ovulation.

Controlled ovarian hyperstimulation in NON-ART cycles (the WHO calls it controlled ovarian stimulation) is defined by the WHO-ICMART as pharmacologic treatment for women in which the ovaries are stimulated to ovulate more than one oocyte. Thus, the goal of COH in NON-ART should be (monthly) multi-follicular development and multiple ovulations. In this definition, NON-ART stands for hyperstimulated cycles besides IVF or ICSI.

Existing Evidence in COH for NON-ART

Why should we stress this difference in approach between COH and OI? Regaining normal ovulatory cycles in women with anovulation, patent tubes, and a partner with normal sperm parameters restores almost normal fertility. Cumulative live birth rates of up to 70% in two years in anovulatory women have been reported (2), almost resembling normal fertility rates. Furthermore, a successful outcome in fertility treatment is defined as the live birth of a healthy singleton. Mono-ovulation is a requirement to achieve this goal.

In COH cycles, the goal is the same: the live birth of a healthy singleton. However, one tries to enhance fertility by releasing two to three oocytes in couples with often a period of unsuccessful mono-ovulation combined with intercourse (unexplained or mild male subfertility, minimal to mild endometriosis) (3) (LOE 1a). Multi-follicular development is one of the keystones for success. It is even questionable whether mono-follicular development in COH cycles increases pregnancy rates. With this strategy, however, one incorporates the chance of achieving a multiple pregnancy, and couples should be informed about these chances beforehand.

Treatment of anovulation with ovulation induction is the subject of Chapters 14 through 21 and will not further be discussed in this chapter.

When to Start COH?

It is obvious that COH is applied in IVF or ICSI cycles. In couples with mild male or unexplained subfertility, it is hypothesized that the subfertility of the couple is related to the subfertility of the woman, and COH in combination with IUI is the most cost-effective first-line treatment option when spontaneous changes are low (4,5) (LOE 1b). By applying COH, one increases the number of available oocytes, improves timing of insemination, and one might correct subtle hormonal imbalances and luteinized unruptured follicle cycles.

But what should we offer couples after 12 ovulatory but unsuccessful OI cycles? What has been proven the most cost-effective treatment option in couples with minimal to mild endometriosis? When should we apply COH in (lesbian) couples or single women using donor sperm?

A large Dutch randomized trial currently investigates whether switching after six ovulatory OI cycles to either IUI of FSH-stimulated cycles improves treatment outcome (M-OVIN study, Netherlands Trial register NTR1449). But further large prospective studies are lacking.

Many centers offer COH (in combination with IUI) after 12 unsuccessful ovulatory cycles suggesting that subfertility is "unexplained" after these 12 cycles. This strategy has not been proven effective, and chances of obtaining a multiple pregnancy are enhanced. On the hand, couples become unmotivated to prolong an unsuccessful treatment option and are often glad to move on. IVF remains their last option but is often not needed.

Once couples are fully informed about chances of success and risks, a balanced decision can be made, a decision, regretfully, not supported by evidence-based guidelines.

Luteal Support?

In COH cycles, using a GNRH agonist or antagonist luteal support is mandatory. But is luteal support also beneficial in OI or non-IVF COH cycles? Lately, there has been a discussion going on regarding luteal support in COH-IUI cycles. The first randomized trials published showed a significant effect of luteal support when gonadotropins are used for COH (LOE 1a) (6). A recent RCT, however, showed no significant effect; thus the end of this discussion has not been reached (LOE 1b) (7). In OI cycles, there seems to be less interest in this subject: Large randomized trials comparing luteal support with placebo on no luteal support in CC cycles are lacking. It has been suggested that the need for luteal support in mono-ovulatory cycles is less pronounced compared to multi-ovulatory cycles (8).

Discussion

It should be clear for both patients and physicians that OI and COH are two different treatment modalities with different goals. Ovulation induction should aim to achieve mono-ovulation and chances to obtain a multiple pregnancy are low. In COH, the ovulation of two to three follicles should be the goal, and multiple pregnancy rates of about 10% are described when strict cancellation criteria are used (5).

Both CC as gonadotropins can be used for OI and COH. In IUI programs, COH with gonadotropins seems more successful (9). Luteal support in mono-ovulatory cycles has not been investigated in randomized trials, and discussion remains ongoing whether luteal support should be advocated in cycles with two to three dominant follicles. Starting support based on small favorable trials only does not seem a cost-effective strategy.

TABLE 12.1

Level of Evidence of Statements

Statement	Level of Evidence
Ovulation induction and controlled ovarian hyperstimulation are two different treatment options and should not be mixed up.	GPP
Controlled ovarian hyperstimulation in non-IVF should aim at achieving two to three follicles.	1a
COH-IUI should be a first-line treatment option in couples with mild male and unexplained subfertility when spontaneous chances of pregnancy are low.	1b
It remains unclear whether luteal support clearly improves cost-effectiveness of COH-IUI cycles.	1a

TABLE 12.2

Grade of Strength for Recommendations

Recommendation	Grade Strength
In couples with mild male or unexplained subfertility, COH-IUI should be a first-line treatment option when spontaneous chances are low.	A
Ovulation induction should result in mono-ovulation, COH in multi-ovulation (two or three dominant follicles).	GPP and A
Luteal support in COH-IUI should only be applied when proven cost-effective.	A

REFERENCES

1. Zegers-Hochschild F, Adamson GD, de Mouzon J, Ishihara O, Mansour R, Nygren K, Sullivan E, van der Poel S. International Committee for Monitoring Assisted Reproductive Technology; World Health Organization. The International Committee for Monitoring Assisted Reproductive Technology (ICMART) and the World Health Organization (WHO) Revised Glossary on ART Terminology, 2009. Hum Reprod. 2009 Nov; 24(11):2683–7.
2. Eijkemans MJ, Imani B, Mulders AG, Habbema JD, Fauser BC. High singleton live birth rate following classical ovulation induction in normogonadotrophic anovulatory infertility (WHO 2). Hum Reprod. 2003 Nov; 18(11):2357–62.
3. van Rumste MM, Custers IM, van der Veen F, van Wely M, Evers JL, Mol BW. The influence of the number of follicles on pregnancy rates in intrauterine insemination with ovarian stimulation: A meta-analysis. Hum Reprod Update. 2008 Nov-Dec; 14(6):563–70.
4. Cohlen BJ, te Velde ER, van Kooij RJ, Looman CW, Habbema JD. Controlled ovarian hyperstimulation and intrauterine insemination for treating male subfertility: A controlled study. Hum Reprod. 1998 Jun; 13(6):1553–8.
5. Bensdorp AJ, Tjon-Kon-Fat RI, Bossuyt PM, Koks CA, Oosterhuis GJ, Hoek A et al. Prevention of multiple pregnancies in couples with unexplained or mild male subfertility: Randomised controlled trial of in vitro fertilisation with single embryo transfer or in vitro fertilisation in modified natural cycle compared with intrauterine insemination with controlled ovarian hyperstimulation. BMJ. 2015 Jan 9; 350:g7771.
6. Miralpeix E, González-Comadran M, Solà I, Manau D, Carreras R, Checa MA. Efficacy of luteal phase support with vaginal progesterone in intrauterine insemination: A systematic review and meta-analysis. J Assist Reprod Genet. 2014 Jan; 31(1):89–100.
7. Hossein Rashidi B, Davari Tanha F, Rahmanpour H, Ghazizadeh M. Luteal phase support in the intra-uterine insemination (IUI) cycles: A randomized double blind, placebo controlled study. J Family Reprod Health. 2014 Dec; 8(4):149–53.
8. Seckin B, Turkcapar F, Yildiz Y, Senturk B, Yilmaz N, Gulerman C. Effect of luteal phase support with vaginal progesterone in intrauterine insemination cycles with regard to follicular response: A prospective randomized study. J Reprod Med. 2014 May-Jun; 59(5-6):260–6.
9. Cantineau AE, Cohlen BJ, Heineman MJ. Ovarian stimulation protocols (anti-estrogens, gonadotrophins with and without GnRH agonists/antagonists) for intrauterine insemination (IUI) in women with subfertility. Cochrane Database Syst Rev. 2007 Apr 18; (2):CD005356.

13

Monitoring of Ovulation Induction Cycles

Kathrin Fleischer

Introduction

Ovulation induction (OI) is frequently applied in anovulatory patients as a first step in infertility treatment. Although OI is highly effective in establishing ovulation, it is, however, not without any risk. There is an ongoing debate on which type of monitoring and which cancelation criteria are best in terms of safety and cost-effectiveness in order to prevent (high-order) multiple pregnancies but maintaining an acceptable pregnancy rate. In this chapter, we describe different methods for monitoring OI in terms of efficacy and safety on the basis of the existing literature. Monitoring OI should help clinicians in predicting (1) the moment of ovulation, (2) inadequate ovarian response, (3) cycles with high risk of multiple pregnancies, and (4) ovarian hyper-response with increased risk of ovarian hyperstimulation syndrome (OHSS).

Overview of Existing Evidence

The size of a follicle with maximum pregnancy competence differs between different types of OI medication. Studies in ovulatory women have observed a larger maximal follicle diameter with clomiphene citrate (mean 20.8 ± 0.7 mm) and letrozole (mean 19.7 ± 0.6 mm) cycles compared with natural cycles (mean 18.2 ± 0.4 mm) (LOE 3). The duration of the follicular phase with clomiphene citrate (CC) was similar to the duration in natural cycles but reduced in cycles with letrozole or gonadotropin (1–3) (LOE 3). Most recent studies propose to administer hCG in the presence of a follicle of 18–22 mm in CC and letrozole cycles and in the presence of a follicle of 17–21 mm in gonadotropin cycles (4,5) (LOE 3).

There is no clear evidence for an endometrium thickness cutoff point in OI cycles. A prospective study on treatment with CC in a mixed population with ovulatory and dysovulatory patients has evaluated the impact of endometrial thickness on pregnancy rates. They found that endometrial thickness was not a predictive factor with a mean thickness of 7.7 ± 0.3 mm in cases of successful pregnancy versus 8.1 ± 0.4 mm in cases of failure (6) (LOE 3). A retrospective study on treatment with gonadotropins has evaluated the impact of endometrial thickness on pregnancy rates and found that a peri-ovulatory endometrial thickness ≥10 mm defined 91% of conception cycles, and no pregnancy occurred when the endometrium measured <7 mm (7) (LOE 3).

In 2006, the Royal College of Obstetricians and Gynaecologists (RCOG) and the National Institute for Clinical Excellence (NICE) both state that ultrasound (US) monitoring is essential during treatment with CC. However, a systematic review of Galazis et al. from 2007 (8) found that there was insufficient evidence to suggest that US monitoring improved pregnancy rates or reduced multiple pregnancy rates. There was, on the other hand, no indication that treatment with CC is safe without US monitoring. No reliable conclusions could be drawn because of the small number of relevant studies and the heterogeneity in the methodology of each study (LOE 1a). In 2013, the NICE guideline (9) advised to offer US monitoring in CC treatment during at least the first cycle of treatment, to ensure a dose that minimizes the risk of multiple pregnancy. Furthermore, the guideline recommended that US monitoring should be an integral part of gonadotropin therapy in order to reduce the risk of multiple pregnancy and the risk of ovarian hyper stimulation (LOE 4).

Although the recruitment of more than one follicle increases the likelihood of pregnancy, it also increases the likelihood of multiple pregnancies. There is a strong link between the number of follicles ≥ 14 mm, the E_2 concentration on the day of hCG/LH surge, and the rate of multiple pregnancies (LOE 3). There is no consensus about cancellation criteria for cycles with a high risk of multiple pregnancies. In CC cycles, the risk of (high-order) multiple pregnancy may be reduced considerably by ultrasound monitoring and cancellation of the cycle if more than two follicles >15 mm diameter are seen (10) (LOE 3). In gonadotropin-induced cycles, a number of studies have analyzed risk factors for multiple pregnancies using US monitoring and determination of serum estradiol concentration (E_2). However, heterogeneity observed in the methodologies of these studies and contradictory results make it difficult to establish strict cancellation criteria or define the most effective and safe method of monitoring. On the basis of the available evidence, a group of experts have reached consensus regarding challenges in polycystic ovary syndrome patients (11). They stated that US is an excellent monitoring method in gonadotropin cycles, and documentation of all follicles greater than 10 mm may be helpful to predict the risk of multiple pregnancies. Furthermore, they proposed to cancel gonadotropin cycles under the age of 38 without any other infertility factor in the presence of more than two follicles ≥ 16 mm or more than one follicle ≥ 16 mm and two additional follicles ≥ 14 mm (11) (LOE 4). Others proposed to use more strict criteria with no more than two follicles ≥ 14 mm with the largest >17 mm (12) (LOE 4). Determination of serum E_2 concentrations could be used to cancel or adjust medication in gonadotropin cycles in order to reduce the risk of multiple pregnancies and OHSS. In the literature, there are no specific cutoff values for E_2 concentrations although some large retrospective trials report E_2 levels <600–1000 pg/ml to prevent (high-order) multiple pregnancies (13) (LOE 3). Other groups stated that monitoring of serum E_2 levels provides no additional information compared with US scan monitoring alone and is therefore not recommended (14) (LOE 3).

Compared with gonadotropin treatment, pulsatile GnRH therapy in WHO 1 anovulation needs little or no monitoring and yields a much higher rate of monofollicular ovulation. Hence, multiple pregnancy rates are very low, and severe OHSS essentially does not occur (10). Also in OI cycles with anti-estrogens, OHSS is a very rare event (LOE 3). The introduction of low-dose FSH protocols for OI has almost completely eliminated the prevalence of severe OHSS. A Cochrane review from 2001 reported an OHSS incidence of 0 - %–7.6% in low- dose FSH protocols; (15) (LOE 1a).

Urinary LH test measurements are a cost-effective and convenient way of ovulation detection at home. Although the overall test accuracy is good, false positive results are possible with high follicular phase LH levels that are present in some PCOS patients. Furthermore, the presence of a LH surge does not always result in ovulation. LH surge configurations can be spiked, biphasic, or plateaued. In women with a regular menstrual cycle, the LH surge duration ranged from 3 to 11 days (16) (LOE 3).

Mid-luteal serum progesterone (P_4) measurement is a well-established method to discover ovulation in retrospect. An elevated level of $P_4 \geq 16$–25 nmol/L in the luteal phase is accepted as proof for ovulation (17). Most live birth–related cycles in oligo- and anovulatory women treated with gonadotropin for OI had even more elevated P_4 levels. Therefore, a mid-luteal P_4 level >31.8 nmol/L may represent a more appropriate threshold for proof of ovulation resulting in live birth. Multiple pregnancies were associated with higher mean mid-luteal P_4 levels (18) (LOE 3).

A menstrual calendar could give additional information because the cycle length may be a relevant indicator of ovulation. Short, that is, <26 days, and long cycles, that is, >35 days, are associated with increased odds of anovulation (19) (LOE 3).

Discussion

There are very few studies restricted to ovulation disorders that compare different monitoring methods in OI with each other. There are no studies on cost-effectiveness in OI monitoring. In order to make the treatment process less invasive, safe, and to minimize costs, US monitoring is currently the most used monitoring method. It is debatable if US should be recommended for monitoring in non-gonadotropin treatment cycles. A strategy could be to monitor the first cycle, and if mono-follicular growth and ovulation is detected, to instruct the patient how to go on without US monitoring. The patient could use a menstrual calendar and urinary LH tests to monitor OI treatment at home. In gonadotropin cycles, US monitoring is compulsory. Adding other methods of monitoring, such as serum E_2 levels, to increase safety and prevent multiple pregnancies is questionable. On the one hand, E_2 measurement adds significantly to costs, and on the other hand, there is growing attention to preventing multiple pregnancies/OHSS with strict cancellation criteria and with mild stimulation protocols. It has to be taken into account that if E_2 detection is used as a monitoring strategy, the reported values in the literature are not universally valid because values depend on the analytical method and the reagent manufacturer. Even when the same kits are used, different laboratories can obtain different results.

Cycle cancellation is advisable if there is no adequate growing follicle on cycle day 20 in CC treatment cycles. The management in gonadotropin cycles depends on the treatment approach. If there is no growing follicle on US, the gonadotropin dosage has to be adjusted until there is growing tendency.

The role of serum P_4 measurement in the luteal phase to confirm ovulation is well established. The disadvantages of this method are its retrospect character, that is, ovulation timing is not possible; its invasiveness; and that it requires an additional visit.

Conclusions

Because of the inhomogeneity of studies, there is not enough evidence to determine which method or combination of methods for OI monitoring should be preferred, particularly with regard to safety and cost-effectiveness. US monitoring is the most frequently used method and could be seen as gold standard for monitoring purposes. It is a quick, efficient and noninvasive way of recording follicular development.

TABLE 13.1

Level of Evidence of Statements

Statement	Level of Evidence
There is insufficient evidence to define which monitoring methods are the most safe and cost-effective. US monitoring is the most advisable method for monitoring in OI.	4
The pregnancy-related diameter of the leading follicle in CC cycles varies between 18 and 22 mm.	3
The pregnancy-related diameter of the leading follicle in gonadotropin cycles varies between 17 and 21 mm.	3
There is insufficient evidence about a pregnancy related cutoff point for endometrium thickness in OI cycles.	3
There is insufficient evidence that US monitoring in CC cycles improves pregnancy rates. There is no sufficient evidence to suggest that US monitoring in CC cycles reduces multiple pregnancy rates.	1a
US monitoring in gonadotropin cycles is mandatory.	4

TABLE 13.2

Grade of Strength for Recommendations

Recommendation	Grade Strength
Vaginal US to monitor follicular growth during ovulation induction is advisable at least in the first treatment cycle when anti-estrogens are used, but it is considered mandatory in all gonadotropin cycles.	GPP
There is no sufficient evidence that US monitoring in CC cycles improves pregnancy rates. There is no sufficient evidence to suggest that US monitoring in CC cycles reduces multiple pregnancy rates.	A
Ovulation induction should only be initiated if patient and physician are prepared to cancel cycles with hyper-response in order to prevent OHSS and multiple pregnancies.	GPP
The pregnancy-related diameter in CC cycles is optimal when the leading follicle reaches 18–22 mm and in gonadotropin cycles when the leading follicle reaches 17–21 mm.	C
In order to avoid multiple pregnancy, achieving mono-follicular or maximal double follicular ovulation is advisable.	GPP
Specific cancellation criteria to prevent multiple pregnancies are recommended, such as no more than two follicles $\geqslant$14 mm, with the largest >17 mm and E_2 concentrations <600–1000 pg/ml.	D
Mid-luteal serum progesterone (P_4) measurement and urinary LH tests are well-established methods to detect ovulation in OI treatment.	D

REFERENCES

1. Jirge PR, Patil RS. Comparison of endocrine and ultrasound profiles during ovulation induction with clomiphene citrate and letrozole in ovulatory volunteer women. Fertil Steril. 2010; 93(1):174–83.
2. Baerwald AR, Walker RA, Randy A, Pierson RA. Growth rates of ovarian follicles during natural menstrual cycles, oral contraception cycles, and ovarian stimulation cycles. Fertil Steril. 2009 Feb; 91(2):440–9.
3. Palatnik A, Strawn E, Szabo A, Robb P. What is the optimal follicular size before triggering ovulation in intrauterine insemination cycles with clomiphene citrate or letrozole? An analysis of 988 cycles. Fertil Steril. 2012 May; 97(5):1089–94.
4. Farhi J, Orvieto R, Gavish O, Homburg R. The association between follicular size on human chorionic gonadotropin day and pregnancy rate in clomiphene citrate treated polycystic ovary syndrome patients. Gynecol Endocrinol. 2010; 26(7):546–8.
5. Shalom-Paz E, Marzal A, Wiser A, Hyman J, Tulandi T. Does optimal follicular size in IUI cycles vary between clomiphene citrate and gonadotrophins treatments? Gynecol Endocrinol. 2014; 30(2):107–10.
6. Kolibianakis EM, Zikopoulos KA, Fatemi HM, Osmanagaoglu K, Evenpoel J, Van Steirteghem A, Devroey P. Endometrial thickness cannot predict ongoing pregnancy achievement in cycles stimulated with clomiphene citrate for intrauterine insemination. Reprod Biomed Online. 2004 Jan; 8(1):115–8.
7. Isaacs JD Jr, Wells CS, Williams DB, Odem RR, Gast MJ, Strickler RC. Endometrial thickness is a valid monitoring parameter in cycles of ovulation induction with menotropins alone. Fertil Steril. 1996 Feb; 65(2):262–6.
8. Galazis N, Zertalis M, Haoula Z, Atiomo W. Is ultrasound monitoring of the ovaries during ovulation induction by clomiphene citrate essential? A systematic review. J Obstet Gynaecol. 2011; 566–71.
9. NICE. Clinical Guideline No.11 Fertility: Assessment and treatment for people with fertility problems. London: National Institute for Clinical Excellence. 2013.
10. Homburg R, Insler V. Ovulation induction in perspective. Hum Reprod Update. 2002 Sep-Oct; 8(5):449–62.
11. Thessaloniki EA-SPCWG. Consensus on infertility treatment related to polycystic ovary syndrome. Fertil Steril. 2008; 89:505–22.
12. Balen AH. Ovulation induction in the management of anovulatory polycystic ovary syndrome. Mol Cell Endocrinol. 2013 Jul; 373(1–2):77–82.
13. Dickey RP. Strategies to reduce multiple pregnancies due to ovulation stimulation. Fertil Steril. 2009 Jan; 91(1):1–17.

14. Hardiman P, Thomas M, Osgood V, Ginasburg J. Are estrogen assays essential for monitoring gonado-trophin stimulant therapy? Gynecol Endocrinol. 1990; 4:261–9.

15. Bayram N, van Wely M, van Der Veen F. Recombinant FSH versus urinary gonadotrophins or recombinant FSH for ovulation induction in subfertility associated with polycystic ovary syndrome. Cochrane Database Syst Rev. 2001; (2): CD002121.

16. Park SJ, Goldsmith LT, Skurnick JH, Wojtczuk A, Weiss G. Characteristics of the urinary luteinizing hormone surge in young ovulatory women. Fertil Steril. 2007 Sep; 88(3):684–90.

17. Fritz MA, Speroff L. Female infertility. In: Speroff L, Fritz MA, editors. Clinical gynecologic endocrinology and infertility. 8th edn. Philadelphia, PA: Lippincott Williams & Wilkins; 2011. Chapter 27.

18. Warne DW, Tredway D, Schertz JC, Schnieper-Samec S, Alam V, Eshkol A. Midluteal serum progesterone levels and pregnancy following ovulation induction with human follicle-stimulating hormone: Results of a combined-data analysis. J Reprod Med. 2011 Jan-Feb; 56(1–2):31–8.

19. Mumford SL, Steiner AZ, Pollack AZ, Perkins NJ, Filiberto AC, Albert PS, Mattison DR, Wactawski-Wende J, Schisterman EF. The utility of menstrual cycle length as an indicator of cumulative hormonal exposure. J Clin Endocrinol Metab. 2012 Oct; 97(10):1871–9.

14

Treatment of WHO 1: GnRH or Gonadotropins?

Cornelis B. Lambalk

Introduction

The administration of gonadotropin releasing hormone (GnRH) given in a very particular episodic way has established itself as the prime therapy for induction of ovulation in hypogonadotropic amenorrhea of supra-pituitary origin (WHO 1). The goal of pulsatile GnRH in ovulation induction is to obtain endogenous pituitary gonadotropin secretion that results in a preferably mono-ovulatory response of the ovaries. So a logical question is why not administer the gonadotropins straight away? In view of current highly advocated evidence-based medical practice lies this relatively straightforward question wide open because the literature provides absolutely insufficient data.

Today, in most leading guidelines, ovulation induction with pulsatile GnRH is mentioned as first in case of WHO 1 anovulation. But evidence levels are, in all situations, graded as low.

A balance has to be made up between the safety, effectiveness, and costs of the GnRH treatment and that of direct treatment with gonadotropins.

Ovulation Induction with Pulsatile GnRH

Indication

The main indication is GnRH deficiency. From the physiological cascade it can be deduced that the primary indication for ovulation induction with pulsatile GnRH is when it must replace the absent or disorderly released endogenous secretagogue. It evidently requires a potentially normal capacity of the pituitary to synthesize and secrete LH and FSH.

Most patients with hypogonadotropic WHO 1 amenorrhea have a supra-pituitary defect resulting in absent or diminished GnRH secretion that varies in severity underlying most other causes of hypogonadotropic amenorrhea, such as in the case of severe stress, weight loss, strenuous exercise, and anorexia nervosa, and variably involve the kisspeptin/neurokinin B system that, in turn, drives the hypothalamic pulse generator. In most cases, the administration of exogenous pulsatile GnRH in a physiological way should restore normal LH and FSH secretion resulting in folliculogenesis, ovulation, and corpus luteum function.

Methodology and Monitoring of Pulsatile GnRH Treatment

GnRH is administered subcutaneously via an infusion pump system that consists of a pod and a remote controller. The pod is filled with the prepared injection fluid; the content is sufficient for 3 days of treatment. After 3 days of use, the pod must be replaced by a new pod.

A suggested practical scenario is each first cycle should be started with a low-pulse dose of 5 μg given with an interval of 120 minutes. This may not result in ovulation, but when it does, it will reduce the "first cycle multiple pregnancy risk" (1). Regardless of whether this first cycle was ovulatory, the pulse dose and/or the pulse frequency should be increased to ensure optimal ovulation induction and luteal function. This is usually the case with a 10-μg pulse every 90 or 120 minutes. Sometimes, higher dosages up to 20 μg are necessary to reach follicular growth. This is, for instance, the case in patients with hypogonadotropic hypogonadism on the basis of a mutation in the GnRH receptor gene, which does not lead to absence, but rather a limited responsiveness of the pituitary (2).

Although the intravenous route of administration is superior to the subcutaneous one in terms of inducing a more physiological pattern of gonadotropin secretion, nowadays only the above-described subcutaneous system is commercially available.

There is no need to adjust the pulse frequency and dose in order to obtain an LH surge. For the occurrence of the surge, GnRH serves as a permissive factor. There is no strict need for ultrasound or laboratory monitoring (LOE 3). A monthly visit, including standard procedures to detect and verify ovulation, suffice. Normally, there is no need for hormonal luteal support treatment.

Under normal circumstances, monitoring of the cycle can be carried out simply by means of a basal body temperature chart during 1 month. When a clear biphasic pattern is observed, ovulation is warranted. Normal luteal function can be verified by judging the length of cycle after the shift in combination with mid-luteal progesterone measurement.

Ovarian and endometrial ultrasound has no additional value.

In the case of pregnancy, treatment can be stopped immediately.

Methodology and Monitoring of Gonadotropin Ovulation Induction

The principle is that of chronic low-dose step-up similar to with ovulation induction in WHO 2 patients with two important differences. In the first place is the type of daily subcutaneous gonadotropin medication that usually requires a combination of FSH and LH activity. The latter, in order to substitute extreme low endogenous LH levels, usually presents in WHO 1 anovulation. By doing so, adequate estrogen secretion by the ovaries is warranted. Second, the starting dose is higher, for example, 150 IU (3).

Otherwise, procedures with regard to follicle growth monitoring cancellation strategies and indication for timing and methods for induction of final maturation and ovulation are identical as with WHO 2 patients with, in addition, hormonal luteal support. For details, see Chapter 17.

Pulsatile GnRH versus Gonadotropins?

Over the past decades, a number of reports appeared describing very good results of pulsatile GnRH treatment in WHO 1 patients with ovulation rates up to 95% per cycle and pregnancy rates around 25% per cycle and reporting cumulative pregnancy rates that varied from 70% during a 3-year time span of registration in a large French study to almost 100% after 6 months in genuine follow-up analysis (Table 14.3).

Reported multiple pregnancy rates vary between 0% and 16.7%. There were no reported OHSS cases. However, the overall LOE is 3.

On the other hand, hardly any recent reports have been published that evaluate the effectiveness and burden of the use of gonadotropins in the WHO 1 patient. Because the gonadotropins act on the ovary directly, high rates of ovulation and pregnancies were reported in older studies but also with high risks of serious complications, such as ovarian hyper stimulation syndrome (OHSS) and higher rates of multiple pregnancies (14.8%–38%) in particular of higher order (Table 14.4). Again, the LOE is 3.

Remarkably, until today, only one relatively small comparative nonrandomized study has been published dating from 1993 (12). There was a nonsignificant higher cumulative conception rate with the pulsatile GnRH and a nonsignificantly lower rate of multiple pregnancies (Table 14.5). The LOE is 3.

TABLE 14.3

Summary of Published Studies Evaluating Pulsatile GnRH in WHO 1 Patients

Author	Patients	Cycles	Ovulation/ Cycle	Pregnancy/ Cycle	Multiple Pregnancy	Cumulative
Berg et al., 1983 (4)	27	40	80%	28%	0%	Not reported
Liu and Yen, 1984 (5)	17	22	86%	41%	Not reported	Not reported
Santoro et al., 1986 (6)	7	20	100%	93%	16.7%	Not reported
Jansen et al., 1987 (7)	27	79	97%	34%	16.7%	88%/six cycles
Blunt and Butt, 1988 (8)	28	84	100%	33%	10%	57%/median of three cycles
Homburg et al., 1989 (9)	118	434	70%	23%	8.8%	93%/6 months
Filicori et al., 1991 (10)	63	105	91%	25%	11%	Not reported
Braat et al., 1991 (11)	34	112	90%	26%	14%	100%/12 months
Martin et al., 1993 (12)	41	118	93%	29%	8.3%	96%/6 months
Filicori et al., 1994 (13)	140	168	81%	20%	5.5%	Not reported
Skarin et al., 1994 (14)	30	96	90%	30%	4.5%	Not reported
Kesrouani et al., 2001 (15)	24	44	100%	46%	0%	83%/18 months
Christin-Maitre et al., 2007 (16)	248	829	Not reported	25%	8.8%	71%/3 years time span evaluation
Total	804	2151	70%–100%	20%–93%	0%–16.7%	

TABLE 14.4

Summary of Studies Evaluating Gonadotropins in WHO 1 Patients

Author	Patients	Cycles	Ovulation/ Cycle	Pregnancy/ Cycle	Multiple Pregnancy	Cumulative
Brown et al., 1969 (3)	45	222	50%	25%	26%	90%/study period
Thompson et al., 1970 (17)	74	257	38%	9%	25%	Not reported
Gemzell, 1975 (18)	15	78	Not reported	27%	19%	Not reported
Oensler et al., 1978 (19)	192	Not reported	Not reported	Not reported	38%	100%/6 cycles
Schwartz et al., 1980 (20)	109	320	95%	30%	27%	73%/14 cycles
Messinis et al., 1988 (21)	50	167	98%	23%	31%	66%/5 years
Martin et al., 1993 (12)	30	111	97%	25%	14.8%	72%/6 months
Carone et al., 2012 (22)	35	70	70%–88%	30%	25%	60%/3 cycles
Total	550	>1225	38%–97%	9%–30%	14.8%–38%	

TABLE 14.5

Summary of Results of the Only Published Study Comparing Gonadotropins and Pulsatile GnRH in WHO 1 Patients

Martin et al., 1993 (12)	Patients	Cycles	Ovulation/ Cycle	Pregnancy/ Cycle	Multiple Pregnancy	Cumulative/ 6 Months
Gonadotropins	30	111	97%	25%	14.8%	72%
Pulsatile GnRH	41	118	93%	29%	8.3%	96%

Discussion

Based on the available literature, it seems that in case of WHO 1 anovulation both pulsatile GnRH and gonadotropin treatment are highly effective with some indication that the physiological pulsatile GnRH is slightly more effective with a lower risk for multiple pregnancy, carries a very low risk for OHSS, allows easy monitoring, and has a low patient burden. Intuitively, it may be more costly, but formal cost-effectiveness studies comparing all mentioned aspects are not available.

Summary

In the clinical practice of ovulation induction, pulsatile treatment with GnRH is of great value in patients with firmly established hypothalamic amenorrhea with cumulative pregnancy rates up to 90% after 12 cycles and should be considered as first choice when the adequate special care that it requires is available. When not available in concert with patient preference, referral to a well-equipped center or ovulation induction with chronic low-dose step-up gonadotropins are the alternative treatment modalities.

TABLE 14.1

Level of Evidence for Statements

Statement	Level of Evidence
One relatively small comparative nonrandomized study showed a nonsignificant higher cumulative conception rate with the pulsatile GnRH and a nonsignificantly lower rate of multiple pregnancies.	3
Case studies show ovulation rate/cycle of 70%–100% and 38%–97% with pulsatile GnRH and gonadotropins, respectively.	3
Case studies show pregnancy rates/cycle of 9%–30% and 20%–93% with pulsatile GnRH and gonadotropins, respectively.	3
Case studies show multiple pregnancy rates of 0%–17% and 15%–38% with pulsatile GnRH and gonadotropins, respectively.	3
Pulsatile GnRH does not require hormonal luteal support treatment.	4
Pulsatile GnRH treatment requires simple once-a-month monitoring for verification of ovulation, resulting in less burden for the patient.	4
Ovarian hyperstimulation is a very rare if not absent side effect of pulsatile GnRH treatment.	4
Most reported side effect is local inflammation at injection site.	4

TABLE 14.2

Grade of Strength for Recommendations

Recommendation	Grade Strength
Treatment with pulsatile GnRH is first choice treatment for ovulation induction for patients with WHO 1 patients with anovulation of supra-pituitary origin.	C/D
Starting dose should be 5 µg per 120 minutes subcutaneously during the first month or first cycle for prevention of multiple pregnancies.	C/D
Standard dose is otherwise 10 µg per 90 minutes.	D
Monitoring requires a once-a-month visit only for verification of ovulation by established means (BBT, mid-luteal progesterone, or ultrasound).	D
When adequate facilities are not available for pulsatile GnRH treatment, patients should be referred.	D
There is urgent need to conduct an adequate randomized controlled cost-effectiveness trial.	D

REFERENCES

1. Lambalk CB, De Koning CH, Braat DD. The endocrinology of dizygotic twinning in the human. Mol Cell Endocrinol. 1998; 145:97–102.
2. Seminara SB, Beranova M, Oliveira LM, Martin KA, Crowley WFJ, Hall JE. Successful use of pulsatile gonadotropin-releasing hormone (GnRH) for ovulation induction and pregnancy in a patient with GnRH receptor mutations. J Clin Endocrinol Metab. 2000; 85:556–62.
3. Brown JB, Evans JH, Adey FD, Taft HP, Townsend L. Factors involved in the induction of fertile ovulation with human gonadotrophins. J Obstet Gynaecol Br Commonw. 1969; 76:289–307.
4. Berg D, Mickan H, Michael S, Döring K, Gloning K, Jänicke F, Rjosk HK. Ovulation and pregnancy after pulsatile administration of gonadotropin releasing hormone. Arch Gynecol. 1983; 233: 205–10.
5. Liu JH, Yen SS. The use of gonadotropin-releasing hormone for the induction of ovulation. Clin Obstet Gynecol. 1984; 27:975–82.
6. Santoro N, Wierman ME, Filicori M, Waldstreicher J, Crowley WF Jr. Intravenous administration of pulsatile gonadotropin-releasing hormone in hypothalamic amenorrhea: Effects of dosage. J Clin Endocrinol Metab. 1986; 62:109–16.
7. Blunt SM, Butt WR. Pulsatile GnRH therapy for the induction of ovulation in hypogonadotropic hypogonadism. Acta Endocrinol Suppl (Copen). 1988; 288:58–65.
8. Jansen RP, Handelsman DJ, Boylan LM, Conway A, Shearman RP, Fraser IS. Pulsatile intravenous gonadotropin-releasing hormone for ovulation-induction in infertile women. I. Safety and effectiveness with outpatient therapy. Fertil Steril 1987; 48:33–8.
9. Homburg R, Eshel A, Armar NA, Tucker M, Mason PW, Adams J, Kilborn J et al. One hundred pregnancies after treatment with pulsatile luteinising hormone releasing hormone to induce ovulation. BMJ. 1989; 25;298(6676):809–12.
10. Filicori M, Flamigni C, Meriggiola MC, Ferrari P, Michelacci L, Campaniello E, Valdiserri A et al. Endocrine response determines the clinical outcome of pulsatile gonadotropin-releasing hormone ovulation induction in different ovulatory disorders. J Clin Endocrinol Metab. 1991; 72:965–72.
11. Braat DD, Schoemaker R, Schoemaker J. Life table analysis of fecundity in intravenously gonadotropin-releasing hormone-treated patients with normogonadotropic and hypogonadotropic amenorrhea. Fertil Steril. 1991; 55:266–71.
12. Martin KA, Hall JE, Adams JM, Crowley WF Jr. Comparison of exogenous gonadotropins and pulsatile gonadotropin-releasing hormone for induction of ovulation in hypogonadotropic amenorrhea. J Clin Endocrinol Metab. 1993; 77:125–9.
13. Filicori M, Flamigni C, Dellai P, Cognigni G, Michelacci L, Arnone R, Sambataro M et al. Treatment of anovulation with pulsatile gonadotropin-releasing hormone: Prognostic factors and clinical results in 600 cycles. J Clin Endocrinol Metab. 1994; 79:1215–50.
14. Skarin G, Ahlgren M. Pulsatile gonadotropin releasing hormone (GnRH)—Treatment for hypothalamic amenorrhoea causing infertility. Acta Obstet Gynecol Scand. 1994; 73:482–5.
15. Kesrouani A, Abdallah MA, Attieh E, Abboud J, Atallah D, Makhoul C. Gonadotropin-releasing hormone for infertility in women with primary hypothalamic amenorrhea. Toward a more-interventional approach. J Reprod Med. 2001; 46:23–8.
16. Christin-Maitre S, de Crécy M. Groupe Français des pompes à GnRH. 2007. [Pregnancy outcomes following pulsatile GnRH treatment: Results of a large multicentre retrospective study]. J Gynecol Obstet Biol Reprod (Paris). 36:8–12.
17. Thompson CR, Hansen LM. Pergonal (menotropins): A summary of clinical experience in the induction of ovulation and pregnancy. Fertil Steril. 1970; 21:844–53.
18. Gemzell C. Induction of ovulation. Acta Obstet Gynaecol Scand Supp. 1975; 47:1–5.
19. Oelsner G, Serr DM, Mashiach S, Blankstein J, Snyder M, Lunenfeld B. The study of induction of ovulation with menotropins: Analysis of results of 1897 treatment cycles. Fertil Steril. 1978; 30:538–44.
20. Schwartz M, Jewelewicz R, Dyrenfurth I, Tropper P, Vande Wiele RL. The use of menopausal and chorionic gonadotropins for induction of ovulation. Sixteen years experience at the Sloane Hospital for Women. Am J Obstet Gynecol. 1980; 138:801–7.

21. Messinis IE, Bergh T, Wide L. The importance of human chorionic gonadotropin support of the corpus luteum during human gonadotropin therapy in women with anovulatory infertility. Fertil Steril. 1988; 50:31–5.
22. Carone D, Caropreso C, Vitti A, Chiappetta R. Efficacy of different gonadotropin combinations to support ovulation induction in WHO type I anovulation infertility: Clinical evidences of human recombinant FSH/human recombinant LH in a 2:1 ratio and highly purified human menopausal gonadotropin stimulation protocols. J Endocrinol Invest. 2012; 35:996–1002.

15

Treatment of WHO 2: Clomiphene Citrate

Roy Homburg and Panagiota Filippou

Introduction

Clomiphene citrate (CC) was first introduced by Greenblatt et al. in 1961 and found to be a safe and efficient way to induce ovulation. The simplicity and inexpensive nature of this treatment have retained CC until today in its position as the first-line treatment for anovulation associated with normal concentrations of endogenous estrogens, (hypothalamic–pituitary dysfunction—WHO Group 2) mainly polycystic ovarian syndrome (PCOS).

By blocking hypothalamic and pituitary estrogen receptors, CC induces a discharge of FSH that is often enough to restore ovulation. Given for 5 days in a dose of 50–150 mg/day, starting from day 2 to 6 of a spontaneous or progestin-induced menstruation, CC will restore ovulation in 73% and induce pregnancy in 36%. Some 20%–25% will not respond at all and are considered to be "clomiphene resistant." The gap between ovulation and pregnancy rates has mainly been attributed to its anti-estrogen effects on endometrium.

As CC blocks the negative feedback mechanism, rising estradiol levels have no effect in stemming the discharge of FSH, and this may invoke multiple follicle development. The risk of multiple gestation is therefore increased and is estimated at about 8%–10% while the singleton live birth rate is reported around 25%.

The prevalence of congenital abnormalities and spontaneous abortion following CC treatment are no different to those seen in spontaneously conceived pregnancies.

Overview of Existing Evidence

Given the well-established effect of CC on ovulation induction and pregnancy outcome, clinical trials have examined a possible improvement in results by adding adjunctive treatments or attempted to establish a potentially superior replacement.

Fields of interest are summarized as follows:

1. CC + Adjunctive treatments
   - CC versus CC + dexamethasone
   - CC versus CC + HCG as ovulation trigger
   - CC versus CC + metformin
2. Comparison between CC and other treatments
   - CC versus placebo
   - CC versus metformin
   - CC versus letrozole
   - CC versus FSH
3. Risk of cancer

In a comparison between CC and a placebo, CC clearly increased the pregnancy rate (OR 9.46, 95% CI 5.1 to 17.7) (1) (LOE 1a).

In order to improve the outcome of treatment with CC, several adjuvants to clomiphene treatment have been suggested.

Clomiphene plus dexamethasone treatment was effective in increasing the pregnancy rate compared to clomiphene alone (1) (LOE 1a). The addition of dexamethasone as an adjunct to clomiphene therapy in a dose of 0.5 mg at bedtime is said to suppress adrenal androgen secretion and induce responsiveness to CC in previous nonresponders, mostly hyperandrogenic women with PCOS and elevated concentrations of dehydroepiandrosterone sulfate (DHEAS). However, glucocorticoid steroid therapy often induces side effects, including increased appetite and weight gain, and should probably be reserved for women who have congenital adrenal hyperplasia as a cause for their anovulation.

The routine addition of hCG at mid-cycle does not improve the conception rates (LOE 1a) (1). In a very powerful randomized control trial (RCT), Legro et al. (2) (LOE 1b), clearly showed the superiority of CC alone over metformin alone (live birth rates 22.5% vs. 7.2%, respectively). Despite this, a couple of recent systematic reviews and meta-analyses of four heterogeneous RCTs found that there was insufficient evidence to establish a difference between metformin and clomiphene citrate in terms of ovulation, pregnancy, live birth, miscarriage, and multiple pregnancy rates in women with PCOS (LOE 1).

No evidence of a difference in effect was found between clomiphene versus tamoxifen (1) (LOE 1a).

Letrozole, the most widely used aromatase inhibitor, is another treatment option for anovulatory PCOS. Aromatase inhibitors have no direct effect on estrogen receptors and therefore do not affect endometrium and do not cause multiple follicular growth. A systematic review including 26 RCTs showed a higher live-birth rate in the letrozole group when letrozole was compared with CC (with or without adjuncts). According to this systematic review, letrozole appears to improve live birth and pregnancy rates in subfertile women with anovulatory PCOS, compared to CC. The quality of this evidence is low, and findings should be regarded with some caution. OHSS was a very rare event with no occurrences in most studies (3) (LOE 1a).

Finally, when comparing CC to low-dose FSH, it appears that pregnancies and live births are achieved more effectively and faster after low-dose FSH, but this result has to be balanced by convenience and cost in favor of CC (4) (LOE 1b).

CC has been thoroughly examined regarding a possible increase in the risk of ovarian cancer. The latest Cochrane database categorically declares that CC does not increase the risk when it is used alone or with gonadotropin (5) (LOE 1a).

Discussion

For the past 50 years, CC has been the first-line treatment for those with absent or irregular ovulation but who have normal basal levels of endogenous estradiol, mainly women with PCOS. It is a cheap, simple, and effective treatment for this population, assuming that there is no additional tubal or male factor. A course of six ovulatory cycles is usually sufficient to know whether pregnancy will be achieved using CC before moving on to more complex treatment as approximately 75% of the pregnancies achieved with CC occur within the first three cycles of treatment. The starting dose is usually 50 mg/day, and it is recommended that 150 mg/day should be the maximum dose as very few pregnancies are achieved at higher doses. An endometrial thickness of less than 7 mm at the time of ovulation due to the anti-estrogen effects of CC, is an adverse prognostic factor (LOE 4). As a result, letrozole has been proposed as a possible replacement of CC, but for the time being, it does not have approval for use in most countries for this indication. CC, on the contrary, is a safe treatment option without adding any risk factor for cancer if it is used in the recommended dose and for no longer than 1 year.

Conclusion

The effectiveness, simplicity, cheap cost, and lack of side effects of CC for anovulatory WHO Group 2 women, mainly with PCOS, makes CC the first option for patients and clinicians. It works well as

TABLE 15.1

Level of Evidence for Statements

Statement	Level of Evidence
CC used for hypothalamic–pituitary dysfunction—WHO Group 2, mainly PCOS, increases ovulation and pregnancy rates compared with placebo.	1a
Clomiphene plus dexamethasone treatment is effective in increasing pregnancy rate compared to clomiphene alone.	1a
The routine addition of hCG in a CC cycle does not improve conception rates.	1a
CC is superior to metformin in achieving live birth in infertile women with PCOS.	1b
Letrozole produces higher live birth and pregnancy rates in subfertile women with anovulatory PCOS, compared to CC.	1a
No evidence of a difference in effect was found between clomiphene versus tamoxifen.	1a
Pregnancies and live births are achieved more effectively and faster after low-dose FSH versus CC for first-line treatment.	1b
There is no convincing evidence of an increase in the risk of ovarian tumors following CC treatment.	1a

TABLE 15.2

Grade of Strength for Recommendations

Recommendation	Grade Strength
CC should be used as first-line treatment to induce ovulation in hypothalamic–pituitary dysfunction—WHO Group 2 women.	A
Even though the addition of dexamethasone as an adjunct to clomiphene therapy increases pregnancy rate, due to its side effects, it should probably be reserved for women who have an adrenal component as a cause for their anovulation.	D
If an anti-estrogen effect on endometrium appears with CC, other treatment options should be considered.	B
The preference of letrozole over CC as first-line treatment in anovulatory PCOS is encouraging (but letrozole is still not licensed for ovulation induction).	A

monotherapy, but in cases of CC resistance or after six ovulatory cycles, the option of other treatments should be considered. Letrozole has so far given promising results and could prove in the future to be a competitor for ovulation induction.

REFERENCES

1. Brown J, Farquhar C, Beck J, Boothroyd C, Hughes E. Clomiphene and anti-oestrogens for ovulation induction in PCOS. Cochrane Database Syst Rev. 2009; (4):CD002249.
2. Legro RS, Barnhart HX, Schlaff WD, Carr BR, Diamond MP, Carson SA, Steinkampf MP et al. Clomiphene, metformin, or both for infertility in the polycystic ovary syndrome. Cooperative Multicenter Reproductive Medicine Network. N Engl J Med. 2007; 356(6):551–66.
3. Franik S, Kremer JA, Nelen WL, Farquhar C. Aromatase inhibitors for subfertile women with polycystic ovary syndrome. Cochrane Database Syst Rev. 2014; (2):CD010287.
4. Homburg R, Hendriks ML, König TE, Anderson RA, Balen AH, Brincat M, Child T et al. Clomiphene citrate or low-dose FSH for the first-line treatment of infertile women with anovulation associated with polycystic ovary syndrome: A prospective randomized multinational study. Hum Reprod. 2012; 27(2):468–73.
5. Rizzuto I, Behrens RF, Smith LA. Risk of ovarian cancer in women treated with ovarian stimulating drugs for infertility. Cochrane Database Syst Rev. 2013; (8):CD008215.

16

Treatment of WHO 2: Aromatase Inhibitors

Anat Hershko Klement and Robert F. Casper

Introduction

Worldwide, approximately 49 million couples have difficulty conceiving, of which about 20 million couples have primary infertility, and 29 million couples have secondary infertility (1). The estimated proportion of patients having an ovulatory disorder out of this population is 15%, most of them classified as WHO class 2 anovulation (PCOS prototype). A simple, safe method of ovulation induction is important because there are millions of women with anovulatory infertility around the world, many without access to ultrasound monitoring or even access to an infertility specialist. An inexpensive, oral agent for ovulation induction that has few side effects and that requires very little if any monitoring to prevent multiple pregnancies is urgently needed. We believe that the use of aromatase inhibitors fulfills these criteria. In this chapter, we describe the use of aromatase inhibitors for ovulation induction in the subset of patients with WHO 2 ovulatory problems.

Overview of Existing Evidence

Letrozole is a potent, nonsteroidal, aromatase inhibitor (AI), originally used for postmenopausal breast cancer therapy, which, at present, is its only registered indication. Unlike the selective estrogen receptor modulators (SERMs), such as clomiphene citrate and tamoxifen, letrozole's mechanism of action does not involve depletion of estrogen receptors nor estrogen receptor antagonism with subsequent anti-estrogenic effects.

Aromatase is the catalyzing enzyme for the rate-limiting step in estrogen biosynthesis. It is expressed in the ovary as well as in other tissues, such as fat, muscle, liver, brain, and breast. Letrozole, a third-generation AI, effectively blocks the production of estrogen from the androgen precursors without disturbing other steroidogenic pathways. Letrozole inhibits the aromatase enzyme by competitively binding to the heme of the cytochrome P450 subunit of the enzyme. Following oral administration, which is not affected by food, letrozole is rapidly absorbed and extensively distributed to tissues. The half-life (t1/2) for letrozole elimination is approximately 2 days. It is metabolized to an inactive metabolite and cleared mostly through renal excretion.

When letrozole was first introduced for ovulation induction, it was hypothesized that it could result in release of the hypothalamic–pituitary axis from estrogenic negative feedback, leading to an increase in gonadotropin secretion and the stimulation of ovarian follicle development. Its relatively short half-life, compared with CC, enables rapid elimination from the body. In addition, because ER downregulation does not occur, no adverse effects on estrogen target tissues are expected.

In the first report of letrozole as a potential ovulation induction agent (2), letrozole was shown to result in successful ovulation in 75% of PCOS patients, and pregnancies were achieved in 25% of them (LOE 3). The initial protocol, which has been most commonly used ever since, included a dose of 2.5 mg on days 3–7 after menses. Since then, accumulated data of randomized clinical trials suggest a clinical pregnancy rate of 32% and a live birth rate of 29.1%. A 5-day versus a 10-day administration protocol for letrozole in the dose of 2.5 mg or increasing the dose to 5 mg or 7.5 mg did not demonstrate a difference in the clinical pregnancy rate (LOE 2a). In early studies, the 2.5 mg daily dose was compared with a 5 mg daily dose in a selected PCOS population, and the results supported a higher number of mature follicles and a higher pregnancy rate for the 5 mg dose (LOE 2b). Comparison to placebo has been rarely performed, for understandable reasons, but the medical literature includes sufficient evidence to support the effectiveness of aromatase inhibitors in terms of ovulation induction efficiency and live birth rates. In particular, there is now high-level evidence (LOE 1a, LOE 1b) that letrozole is more effective than clomiphene citrate in ovulation induction and clinical and live birth rates in PCOS patients (but letrozole is still not licensed for ovulation induction) (3,4). The latest multicenter clinical trial addressed this question by randomly assigning 750 women, in a 1:1 ratio, to receive letrozole or clomiphene citrate for up to five treatment cycles. The cumulative ovulation rate was significantly higher with letrozole than with clomiphene citrate (61.7% of treatment cycles vs. 48.3%, respectively, <0.001), and the risk ratio for live birth was 1.44 in favor of letrozole (95% confidence interval, 1.10 to 1.87). A meta-analysis surveying nine clinical randomized trials summarized birth rates for letrozole compared to clomiphene citrate followed by timed intercourse. The birth rate was higher in the letrozole group (OR 1.64, 95% CI 1.32 to 2.04, *n* = 1783, LOE 1a).

Even when used in a PCOS population with significant resistance to clomiphene citrate (failed ovulation after six cycles, up to 150 mg/day), a 54.6% response rate was achieved with letrozole, and out of these cycles, 25% resulted in conception. No specific characteristics were found to differentiate the letrozole responsive group in terms of age, period of infertility, body mass index (BMI), waist or hip circumference, waist/hip ratio, LH, FSH, or LH/FSH ratio (LOE 3).

Other alternatives for ovulation induction include ovarian drilling and gonadotropin injections. Naturally, most comparisons of letrozole to these other options were performed in a population of PCOS patients who were either resistant to clomiphene citrate or failed to conceive because of anti-estrogen adverse effects. No differences were observed in the clinical pregnancy rates or live birth rates when letrozole was compared to ovarian drilling (LOE 1a). In a heterogeneous patient population that failed at least one clomiphene citrate treatment, letrozole achieved comparable pregnancy rates to continuous injectable gonadotropins for ovulation induction (LOE 1b). Among individuals who failed to conceive with less than three cycles of clomiphene citrate and whose medications were changed because of thin uterine lining (anti-estrogenic side effect) or intolerable symptomatic side effects, the average pregnancy rates per cycle for letrozole use alone and for gonadotropin treatment alone were equivalent (LOE 1b). Specifically for patients with three failed clomiphene citrate cycles, treatment with gonadotropins starting cycle day 3 was compared to a combination of letrozole 2.5 mg between days 3 and 7, followed by gonadotropins starting on cycle day 5. The addition of letrozole significantly decreased total gonadotropin dose and number of days to ovulation induction without any adverse effects on endometrial thickness. Mono-ovulation was achieved in the letrozole-treated women with equivalent pregnancy rates to gonadotropin stimulation (LOE 2a). In summary, the simple oral use of a low-cost medication was determined to be at least equivalent in success to either an invasive surgical procedure or an expensive injectable medication. In the case of gonadotropins, multiple pregnancies are another concern that may also be obviated by letrozole use.

After choosing to use letrozole for ovulation induction, there are still a few treatment protocol decisions that need to be considered. First, is there a need for endometrial shedding before treatment initiation? The literature for clomiphene citrate suggests that conception and live birth rates are lower in women with PCOS after a spontaneous menses or progestin-induced withdrawal bleed as compared to anovulatory cycles without progestin withdrawal (LOE 1b). We believe the best explanation for this finding relates to the estrogen receptor (ER) depletion by clomiphene citrate that may result in poor endometrial growth and development. If there is no endometrial shedding and the endometrium is already near the acceptable thickness needed for implantation at the time clomiphene citrate is introduced, then the ER depletion effect may be less problematic. Because the mechanism of action of letrozole does not involve any ER antagonist activity, it is unlikely that shedding will have a deleterious effect on the cycle outcome. To the best of our knowledge, there is not a published study addressing this question solely for patients undergoing letrozole treatment.

Other relevant issues in the use of letrozole for ovulation induction cycles include the following questions: Is there a need for hCG triggering? What is the ideal follicular size on the day of hCG triggering? Is there any added value of IUI in cases of a normal sperm count? What is the need for progesterone luteal support? The literature provides little if any evidence to help with these questions. However, there is limited data that demonstrates a higher pregnancy rate in PCOS patients who were triggered to ovulate by hCG in letrozole-induced cycles (LOE 3). Higher pregnancy rates were achieved when the leading follicles were in the 23 to 28 mm range (LOE 3). Compared to timed intercourse, the addition of IUI to letrozole induction of ovulation does not seem to increase the pregnancy rate in couples with PCOS and normal semen analysis (LOE 3). There is low-quality evidence for higher clinical pregnancy rates (LOE 3) in women with PCOS who used letrozole for ovulation induction when intra-vaginal progesterone luteal support was provided.

Due to its mode of action, letrozole is not expected to result in ovarian hyperstimulation syndrome (OHSS), especially in the case of ovulation induction that is not followed or combined with gonadotropins; indeed there are no reports of OHSS cases in letrozole ovulation induction cycles. When all embryos are frozen to reduce the risk of OHSS in overstimulated IVF cycles, it is possible that the use of letrozole in the luteal phase may further reduce the risk by lowering estrogen concentrations (LOE 1b).

The multiple pregnancy rate in letrozole cycles in PCOS patients is 0.7% (LEO 1a) and is significantly lower than the rate in clomiphene citrate cycles (1.8, 95% CI 0.17–0.84, LOE 1a). The reduced rate of multiples in terms of pregnancies was supported by Legro et al. in their latest 2014 study addressing letrozole versus clomiphene although this was a secondary outcome measure and did not reach a statistical significance (RR 0.46, 95% CI 0.13–1.58, $P = 0.32$). This reflects the physiology and pharmacology of the medication. Aromatase inhibitors do not deplete estrogen receptors in the brain. Once the patient stops taking letrozole on cycle day 7, the dominant follicle grows and estrogen levels rise, resulting in a normal negative central feedback on FSH levels. Suppression of FSH by estrogen leads to atresia of the smaller growing follicles and eventually to a mono-follicular ovulation in most cases. Multiple pregnancies are high risk with a higher maternal morbidity and higher prematurity rates, resulting in neonatal complications and a higher cost to the health care system. Therefore, a substantial advantage of letrozole, and another pivotal consideration in its use as a primary treatment for PCOS, is the reduced risk of multiple pregnancies with less need for monitoring. We should be mindful that regardless of high-order pregnancies, PCOS is associated with increased risk of pregnancy complications, such as gestational diabetes, gestational hypertension, and preeclampsia.

Pregnancy outcomes in terms of fetal anomaly rates are a great concern with any infertility treatment. In a multicenter Canadian study including 911 babies (5), overall congenital malformations and chromosomal abnormalities were 14 of 514 babies in the letrozole group (2.4%) and 19 of 397 babies in the CC group (4.8%). The major malformation rate in the letrozole group was 1.2% (six of 514) and in the CC group was 3.0% (12 of 397). These differences in rates were not statistically significant. However, seven newborns in the CC group (1.8%) and one in the letrozole group (0.2%) had congenital cardiac anomalies ($P = 0.02$). The miscarriage rate is not different in clomiphene citrate and letrozole ovulation induction cycles (LOE 1a).

Discussion

Current experimental literature and clinical experience support the use of letrozole as a primary agent for ovulation induction in WHO class 2 ovulatory disorder due to its higher ovulation rates compared to clomiphene citrate and its superiority in terms of live birth. Because of this extensive experience in ovulation induction, letrozole is now being tested for other fertility indications involving its possible beneficial influence on endometrial receptivity in ART cycles. Letrozole has been demonstrated to be equal to ovarian drilling and gonadotropin administration in terms of live birth rates. Because these alternative therapeutic options are either invasive or involve a substantial cost and potential for complications, letrozole stands out as a simple, practical, and affordable option among available treatments for ovulation induction. Its safety profile is reassuring in terms of low multiple pregnancy rates, lack of OHSS, and low fetal anomaly rates. Other supportive considerations for its use include its oral route of administration,

TABLE 16.1

Level of Evidence of Statements

Statement	Level of Evidence
Ovulation induction for PCOS patients with letrozole compared to clomiphene citrate (followed by timed intercourse) results in a significantly higher live birth rate for letrozole treatment.	1a
In a clomiphene citrate–resistant PCOS population, letrozole results in a comparable live birth rate to ovarian drilling.	1a
After a clomiphene failure in more than one cycle, for the purpose of ovulation induction, pregnancy rates are equivalent for letrozole versus gonadotropin injections.	1b
Higher pregnancy rates are achieved when the leading follicles are in the 23 to 28 mm range for letrozole ovulation induction cycles.	3
Compared to timed intercourse, IUI does not seem to increase the pregnancy rate in couples with PCOS and normal semen analysis treated with letrozole for ovulation induction.	3
Vaginal progesterone luteal support after letrozole ovulation induction may result in a higher clinical pregnancy rate in women with PCOS.	3

TABLE 16.2

Grade of Strength for Recommendations

Recommendation	Grade Strength
Letrozole is the treatment of choice for ovulation induction in PCOS patients (but letrozole is still not licensed for ovulation induction).	A
Letrozole is the treatment of choice in cases of clomiphene resistance or clomiphene failure.	A

low cost (in Canada, $0.50 per 2.5 mg tablet for generic letrozole), relatively short half-life, and negligible side effects. Common practice involves a dose of 2.5 mg on days 3–7 following a spontaneous or induced period. There is a lack of sufficient evidence to recommend a higher dose although this may facilitate a better response and outcome rates in some patients. Letrozole seems therefore the best first-line treatment option in lean women with WHO2 anovulation as well as in women with PCOS. In overweight or obese women, it constitutes the best second-line treatment option after lifestyle modification leading to weight loss.

REFERENCES

1. Mascarenhas, MN, Flaxman SR, Boerma T, Vanderpoel S, Stevens GA. National, regional, and global trends in infertility prevalence since 1990: A systematic analysis of 277 health surveys. PLoS Med. 2012; 9(12):e1001356.
2. Mitwally, MF, Casper RF. Use of an aromatase inhibitor for induction of ovulation in patients with an inadequate response to clomiphene citrate. Fertil Steril. 2001, Feb; 75(2):305–9.
3. Legro, RS, Zhang H, Nichd Reproductive Medicine Network Eunice Kennedy Shriver. Letrozole or clomiphene for infertility in the polycystic ovary syndrome. N Engl J Med. 2014, Oct; 371(15):1463–4.
4. Franik, S, Kremer JA, Nelen WL, Farquhar C. Aromatase inhibitors for subfertile women with polycystic ovary syndrome. Cochrane Database Syst Rev. 2014; 2:CD010287.
5. Tulandi, T, Martin J, Al-Fadhli R, Kabli N, Forman R, Hitkari J, Librach C et al. Congenital malformations among 911 newborns conceived after infertility treatment with letrozole or clomiphene citrate. Fertil Steril. 2006, Jun; 85(6):1761–5.

17

Treatment of WHO 2: Insulin Sensitizers

Lisa J. Moran, Marie Misso, Helena J. Teede, and Jacqueline Boyle

Introduction

Affecting 12%–18% of women, depending on diagnostic criteria and population studied, polycystic ovary syndrome (PCOS) is prevalent and underrecognized with serious health impacts for affected women and their families. PCOS is the principal cause of anovulatory female infertility and increases the risk of pregnancy complications, such as miscarriage, fetal anomalies, preeclampsia, and gestational diabetes. PCOS is also associated with a range of metabolic features, which include obesity, metabolic syndrome, type 2 diabetes, and cardiovascular risk factors. PCOS is underpinned by insulin resistance. Obesity, more common in PCOS, increases the prevalence and severity of PCOS by exacerbating insulin resistance. Insulin resistance with compensatory hyperinsulinemia affects up to 85% of women with PCOS. Hyperinsulinemia leads to higher ovarian androgen biosynthesis and decreased hepatic sex hormone binding globulin (SHBG) synthesis. The increased local ovarian androgen production augmented by hyperinsulinemia causes premature follicular atresia and anovulation with insulin having reproductive hormonal effects. The contribution of insulin resistance to anovulation in PCOS has led to the introduction of insulin-sensitizing agents as a pharmacological therapy to potentially induce ovulation and enhance fertility. Of the insulin-sensitizing agents, metformin has been most widely studied in women with PCOS since 1994 and has the most reassuring safety profile (1). Metformin is a biguanide, used as an oral antihyperglycemic agent for the prevention and management of type 2 diabetes and is available in two formulations: immediate and extended release (2).

Overview of Existing Evidence

A recent search of the literature revealed that there were more than 150 randomized controlled trials and systematic reviews addressing the use of metformin for various indications of PCOS (2). In this setting, opinions about metformin use in PCOS are often based on small, poor-quality studies, many of which are inappropriate for use in clinical decision making. Evidence-based guidelines that synthesize this evidence and use a clinical judgment process to provide recommendations for the use of metformin in women with PCOS include the rigorously developed PCOS Australian Alliance evidence-based guideline for assessment and management of PCOS and the U.S. Endocrine Society guideline. Effect sizes and measures of heterogeneity provided here are from exemplar systematic review evidence included in the PCOS Australian Alliance; however, the discussion incorporates the broad body of evidence.

Metformin has been shown to be better than placebo for ovulation rate and pregnancy rate in women with PCOS; however, there was significant statistical heterogeneity in much of the analyses. In women with PCOS and with a BMI ≤ 30 kg/m^2 ($p = 0.00071$); with a BMI ≥ 30 kg/m^2 ($p = 0.0073$), and in women who were clomiphene citrate sensitive or had unknown clomiphene citrate sensitivity ($p = 0.000019$), metformin was better than placebo for ovulation rate. There was no benefit of metformin over placebo in women with PCOS who were clomiphene citrate resistant. Metformin maintained superiority over placebo when all women were combined; however, there was significant statistical heterogeneity in this group ($I^2 = 69\%$) and in those with a BMI ≤30 kg/m^2 ($I^2 = 88\%$). Metformin outperformed placebo for pregnancy rate in women with PCOS and a BMI ≤30 kg/m^2 ($p = 0.000017$) with little statistical heterogeneity ($I^2 = 40\%$), but no difference was noted in those with BMI ≥30 kg/m^2, in clomiphene citrate naïve women, women who were clomiphene citrate resistant, or women who were clomiphene citrate sensitive or had unknown clomiphene citrate sensitivity. Combined analyses of all women demonstrated a benefit of metformin over placebo ($p < 0.00001$) without statistical heterogeneity for pregnancy rate.

Based on limited data that extended to study live birth rates, no difference between metformin and placebo for live birth rate or miscarriage rate has been noted. Metformin induced more minor gastrointestinal-related adverse events compared to placebo ($p < 0.00001$) with little statistical heterogeneity ($I^2 = 25\%$) (3). Metformin therefore improves ovulation and pregnancy rate, but there is currently inadequate data for an effect on live birth rates. The majority of studies used 1500–2000 mg per day of metformin, and most did not use extended release. It is generally recommended if using metformin that doses are initiated at 500 mg daily and increased by 500 mg daily every 2 weeks. There is considerable controversy over when metformin should be ceased if pregnancy occurs. In general, there is inadequate evidence to support continuing metformin following conception with more research needed. With regards to time to ovulation with metformin, most of the published research is of 6 months duration with ovulation commencing relatively early in this time but with no data on a mean or median time to ovulation currently available. Regular menses are also generally reported by 3 months and continue to improve with time unrelated to pregnancy or ovulation.

Metformin has been compared to and combined with other ovulation-induction agents and methods with uncertain benefit. Disagreement across studies measuring the same comparisons and outcomes is reflected in statistical heterogeneity. Metformin was associated with a reduced ovulation rate ($p < 0.00001$) and pregnancy rate ($p = 0.018$) compared to clomiphene citrate in women with PCOS and in those with a BMI ≥30 kg/m^2 ($p < 0.00001$ and $p = 0.00001$, respectively); however, there was little difference in ovulation rate in those with a BMI ≤30 kg/m^2 (significant statistical heterogeneity, $I^2 = 78\%$ and 91%, respectively). There was no benefit of metformin over clomiphene citrate for live birth rate, and clomiphene citrate was better than metformin for live birth rate in those with a BMI ≥30 kg/m^2 ($p = 0.00002$) (without statistical heterogeneity). There was no difference in multiple pregnancy rate or miscarriage rate (3). Metformin therefore did not result in improved reproductive outcomes compared to clomiphene citrate.

Metformin plus clomiphene citrate was better than clomiphene citrate alone for ovulation rate in women with PCOS ($p < 0.00001$), including subgroup analysis in those with a BMI ≤30 kg/m^2 ($p = 0.009$), with a BMI ≥30 kg/m^2 ($p < 0.00001$), with clomiphene citrate resistance ($p < 0.00001$), and in those with unknown clomiphene citrate sensitivity ($p < 0.00001$). There was significant statistical heterogeneity for all subgroups except women with clomiphene citrate resistance. There was no difference in those with clomiphene citrate–sensitive PCOS. Pregnancy rates were better with combined metformin plus clomiphene citrate than with clomiphene citrate alone ($p = 0.006$), including subgroups of women with a BMI ≥30 kg/m^2 ($p = 0.004$), clomiphene citrate naïve women ($p < 0.0001$), and women with clomiphene citrate resistance ($p = 0.0001$). There was significant statistical heterogeneity for all subgroups except in those with a BMI ≥30 kg/m^2 (little heterogeneity $I^2 = 40\%$) and those with clomiphene citrate resistance. There was no difference in those with a BMI ≤30 kg/m^2 and in those who were clomiphene sensitive or with unknown clomiphene citrate sensitivity. Metformin plus clomiphene citrate was better than clomiphene citrate alone for live birth rate in women with clomiphene citrate resistance ($p = 0.03$ without statistical heterogeneity). Live birth rate was similar between the two groups in those with a BMI ≤30 kg/m^2, a BMI ≥30 kg/m^2, and in those with clomiphene citrate naïve PCOS as well as when subgroups were combined. There was no difference between the interventions for miscarriage rate and multiple pregnancy rate, and clomiphene citrate alone had fewer gastrointestinal-related adverse events (3). Metformin and clomiphene citrate in combination therefore provided benefits for ovulation and pregnancy rates, particularly in women with a BMI >30 kg/m^2.

Metformin plus clomiphene citrate was better than metformin alone for ovulation rate, pregnancy rate, and live birth rate in women with PCOS ($p < 0.0001$ for all three outcomes, no significant heterogeneity). There was no difference for miscarriage rate or adverse events (3).

These findings have been translated to evidence-based clinical practice recommendations (see Table 17.2). It is also important to note that intensive lifestyle modification is recommended first line in overweight women before any pharmacological therapy for infertility management (Table 17.1; see also Chapter 20). Current evidence-based guidelines recommend intensive lifestyle modification, particularly in those with a BMI ≥30 kg/m^2, including frequent multidisciplinary engagement for 3 to 6 months as first-line therapy (LOE 1b) (3). This recommendation was underpinned by randomized controlled trials, which found that there was no benefit of metformin over lifestyle (2,3). Long-term studies in the general population and in people with diabetes suggest that metformin could enhance the effectiveness of lifestyle modification for fertility outcomes; however, at present, there is an absence of large-scale studies in the PCOS setting.

Discussion

There remains little certainty and much controversy on the role of metformin for anovulation in PCOS despite the abundance of randomized controlled trials (RCTs) and systematic reviews addressing the use of metformin in isolation or in conjunction with other pharmacotherapies in PCOS. Opinions about metformin use in women with PCOS are often derived from small, poor-quality studies, which are inappropriate for guiding clinical decision making and, when pooled in meta-analysis, provide heterogeneous and thus clinically challenging findings.

Evidence-based guidelines that consider evidence as well as clinical judgment provide support for the use of the following:

- Clomiphene citrate over metformin based on efficacy
- Metformin combined with clomiphene citrate
- Metformin in combination with clomiphene citrate in women with PCOS who have not responded to clomiphene citrate as first-line therapy either in terms of ovulation or pregnancy

There is evidence that the use of metformin may be associated with mild gastrointestinal-related adverse events, and therefore, women with PCOS who are prescribed metformin (alone or in combination with clomiphene citrate) to improve fertility outcomes should be informed about associated gastrointestinal-related side effects. The risk of multiple pregnancy is also increased with clomiphene citrate use (5%–8%), and therefore, monitoring is recommended (3). This was identified as a clinical practice point and was developed by the clinical guideline development group based on discussion of clinical concerns in management. Specific recommendations on monitoring were not made as this question was not the subject of specific evidence synthesis and review. Monitoring approaches vary but include the use of ultrasound during treatment to detect multiple follicular development and potentially estradiol levels, which can guide clinicians on when to cancel the cycle if risks of multiple pregnancy are too high. In many countries, the use of ovulation induction agents are restricted to experienced reproductive endocrinologists or fertility specialists to optimize awareness of risk, monitoring, and prevention.

Conclusions

Despite the large body of evidence comparing the insulin sensitizer metformin with control/placebo, lifestyle interventions, and clomiphene citrate, its use for ovulation induction in women with PCOS remains uncertain. Metformin has a limited role for ovulation induction for fertility in PCOS until large, high-quality studies are conducted that include women across the BMI range.

TABLE 17.1

Level of Evidence for Statements

Statement	Level of Evidence
Metformin should not be first-line therapy for ovulation induction and should not be commenced until intensive lifestyle modification has been attempted.	1b

TABLE 17.2

Grade of Strength for Recommendations

Recommendation	Grade Strength
Pharmacological ovulation induction should not be recommended for first-line therapy in women with polycystic ovary syndrome who are morbidly obese (body mass index ≥ 35 kg/m^2) until appropriate weight loss has occurred either through diet, exercise, bariatric surgery, or other appropriate means.	C
Metformin could be used alone to improve ovulation rate and pregnancy rate in women with polycystic ovary syndrome who are anovulatory, have a body mass index ≤ 30 kg/m^2, and are infertile with no other infertility factors.	B
If one is considering using metformin alone to treat women with polycystic ovary syndrome who are anovulatory, have a body mass index ≥ 30 kg/m^2, and are infertile with no other infertility factors, clomiphene citrate should be added to improve fertility outcomes.	A
Metformin should be combined with clomiphene citrate to improve fertility outcomes rather than persisting with further treatment with clomiphene citrate alone in women with polycystic ovary syndrome who are clomiphene citrate resistant, anovulatory, and infertile with no other infertility factors.	A

REFERENCES

1. Palomba S, Falbo A, Zullo F, Orio FJ. Evidence-based and potential benefits of metformin in the polycystic ovary syndrome: A comprehensive review. Endocr Rev. 2009; 30:1–50.
2. Misso ML, Teede HJ. Metformin in women with PCOS, CONS. Endocrine. 2014; 48:428–33.
3. Teede HJ, Misso ML, Deeks AA, Moran LJ, Stuckey BG, Wong JL, Norman RJ et al. Assessment and management of polycystic ovary syndrome: Summary of an evidence-based guideline. Med J Aust. 2011; 195:S65–112.

18

Treatment of WHO 2: Laparoscopic Electrocautery of the Ovaries

Saad Amer, Neriman Bayram, and Marleen Nahuis

Introduction

Polycystic ovary syndrome (PCOS) is the most frequent cause of WHO II anovulation affecting ~10% of women of reproductive age. In 1935, Stein and Leventhal were the first to describe the association between polycystic ovaries (seen at laparotomy) and menstrual irregularities, sterility, hirsutism, and obesity. They performed laparotomies on a group of these patients to obtain ovarian biopsies for diagnostic purposes. Unexpectedly, they observed postoperative resumption of regular menses and fertility in most of their patients. Surgical ovarian wedge resection (OWR) was therefore established as the first effective treatment for anovulatory PCOS patients with high success rates (80% resumption of regular menses and ~60% conception). In the 1960s, OWR was largely abandoned (due to its associated morbidity) in favor of the newly introduced clomiphene citrate, which became the standard first-line ovulation induction therapy in PCOS. In the late 1960s and with the development of minimal invasive surgery, there was a renewed interest in surgical ovulation induction carried out laparoscopically. In 1967, Palmer and De Brux in France and Steptoe in Great Britain were the first to describe laparoscopic ovarian biopsy in PCOS women. However, this new approach did not find its way to clinical practice possibly due to the limited number of centers performing laparoscopic surgery, which was still in its early days. In 1984, Gjönnaess published the first study on laparoscopic electrocautery of the ovary (LEO) reporting very encouraging success rates (91% ovulation rate). Following this publication, LEO gained much popularity worldwide, and a plethora of studies has since been published confirming its efficacy and safety. The underlying mechanisms of LEO actions remain largely uncertain. Several hypotheses have been postulated, such as removal of a mechanical barrier to ovulation or decreased ovarian androgen synthesis due to thermal tissue destruction. Whatever the mechanism may be, it is evident that a small amount of damage to ovarian tissue seems to restore the ovulatory cycle in a high proportion of patients.

Overview of Existing Evidence

This review presents the available evidence for LEO in anovulatory PCOS patients focusing mainly on the following clinically important issues:

- The current role of LEO
- Techniques of LEO
- The optimum number of punctures during LEO
- The optimal depth of needle insertion into the ovary
- Long-term effects and safety of LEO

The Current Role of LEO

As clomiphene citrate (CC) is a relatively cheap, simple, effective, and safe treatment, it is widely regarded as the standard first-line treatment for ovulation induction in anovulatory PCOS women (LOE 2). When LEO was compared in an RCT to CC as a first-line treatment in anovulatory PCOS, it was not found to offer any advantages over CC. It was therefore concluded that LEO should not be offered as a first-line treatment in PCOS (LOE 1b) (1).

In PCOS women with CC resistance, defined as failure to ovulate on the maximum dose (150 mg/ day) or failure to conceive despite regular ovulation, the choice is between LEO and gonadotrophin therapy. Both these modalities are equally effective in inducing ovulation and generating pregnancies (LOE 1a) (2,3). A recent Cochrane systematic review compared the outcome of LEO with various medical agents used for ovulation induction in PCOS women, including clomiphene citrate (CC) alone or CC plus tamoxifen, gonadotrophins, and aromatase inhibitors. The review found no significant differences in live birth rates between LEO and medical ovulation induction. However, LEO was associated with lower multiple pregnancy rates. Furthermore, the cost per live birth achieved with LEO has been estimated to be 22% lower than that achieved with gonadotrophin therapy (LOE 1b). A long-term economic evaluation study reported a saving of €3,220 (~20%) per live birth when a strategy starting with LEO before gonadotrophins was adopted (4). LEO should therefore be considered the second-line treatment of choice in preference to gonadotrophin therapy in CC-resistant PCOS women (LOE 1a) (2). LEO has also been recommended in gonadotrophin-over-respondent PCOS women (LOE 2).

Techniques of LEO

Numerous techniques of laparoscopic ovarian surgery to induce ovulation in PCOS women have been developed over the years. Most of the techniques involve either taking ovarian biopsies or making multiple punctures on the surface of the ovary using monopolar or bipolar electrocoagulation or laser. Comparing these three energy modalities, bipolar electrocoagulation seems to result in more destruction per burn when applied to fresh bovine ovaries (LOE 2). More recently, there have been several attempts to use a transvaginal route to perform the ovarian surgery, utilizing either a fertiloscopy or an ultrasound-guided approach.

Currently, the two most commonly used techniques for LEO are monopolar laparoscopic ovarian drilling (LOD) and bipolar electrocautery. Both approaches are widely accepted due to their relative simplicity, effectiveness, safety, and low costs (LOE 2). In both techniques, the utero-ovarian ligament is grasped with atraumatic grasping forceps, and the ovary is lifted up and stabilized in position to avoid thermal injury to the bowel. In LOD, a laparoscopic monopolar diathermy needle is used to penetrate the ovarian capsule at a number of points. The active distal part of the needle should measure 7–8 mm in length and 2 mm in diameter and project from an insulated solid cone with a wider diameter. When the needle penetrates the capsule of the ovary, the insulated cone controls the depth of penetration and minimizes thermal damage to the ovarian surface. The needle should be applied to the anti-mesenteric surface of the ovary at a right angle to avoid slippage and to minimize surface damage. After insertion of the needle, 30-watt monopolar coagulation electricity current is activated for 5 seconds. One should be aware that electricity activated before penetrating the surface of the ovary could cause charring of the ovarian surface. However, it may be necessary to facilitate the needle insertion by a short burst of diathermy. In bipolar electrocoagulation, a bipolar insulated needle electrode (length 345 mm, diameter 5 mm) is pressed at a right angle to an ovarian follicle, and the needle (length 15 mm, shaft 0.9 mm) is inserted in the follicle and surrounding tissue. Each ovary can be punctured randomly five to 10 times, depending on its size. The automatic stop function guarantees a reproducible coagulation. In both mono- and bipolar techniques, the site of application should be away from the ovarian hilum and the fallopian tube. This is necessary to avoid damage of the hilum (which can lead to ovarian atrophy) and the fallopian tube (which can cause mechanical infertility).

How Much Energy Should Be Used for LEO?

The amount of thermal energy used and number of punctures made in each ovary varied considerably in different studies. Between 3 and 25 punctures have been reported with power settings between 30 and 400 w. The only technique that has been investigated for the optimum amount of thermal energy is monopolar LOD. In a retrospective review of 161 women who underwent LOD, 3 punctures (450 joules/ovary) seemed to represent the optimum amount of energy above which no further improvement of the outcome could be achieved (LOE 2). In a prospective dose-finding study utilizing an "up-and-down design" and involving 30 women with anovulatory PCOS undergoing LOD, four punctures per ovary at 30 w for 5 seconds (600 joules) per puncture were found to represent the optimum number required to achieve the best result (LOE 2) (5). Unilateral LEO has been reported in different controlled trials to be as efficacious as bilateral LEO, but the evidence is not conclusive, and long-term data are lacking.

Depth of Needle Insertion into the Ovary

Deep insertion of the needle into the ovarian stroma during LEO has been deemed necessary to achieve optimal results with minimal thermal energy (LOE 2). The rationale for this approach is that deep penetration allows the delivery of thermal energy to the ovarian stroma thereby directly destroying androgen producing tissue (LOE 2) (6). Deep penetration also helps to avoid ovarian surface charring, which is a cause of postoperative adhesion formation. The theoretical benefits of deep needle insertion has been supported by several studies, which showed that a needle insertion of about 8 mm into ovarian stroma results in good clinical outcome with a relatively small amount of energy (LOE 2) (6). On the other hand, studies applying shallow craters of 2–4 mm depth on the ovarian surface required a very high amount of thermal energy (>3750 joules/ovary) to achieve successful outcomes (6).

Long-Term Effects of LEO

There have been several studies evaluating the long-term effects of LEO, all consistently reporting long-lasting beneficial reproductive and endocrine effects in up to 50% of women undergoing this procedure (LOE 2). However, there is now emerging literature evidence that women with PCOS tend to resume regular menstrual cycles with advancing age. It is therefore possible that the favorable late reproductive effects observed in various studies could have been the effect of advancing age rather than LEO. In order to investigate this further, a longitudinal cohort study compared the long-term clinical outcome of women with anovulatory PCOS who underwent LEO ($n = 116$) with that of a matched group of PCOS women ($n = 38$) who did not undergo LEO. The study showed that LEO contributed significantly to the long-term endocrine and clinical improvements in PCOS women (LOE 2) (7).

Another longitudinal cohort study compared the long-term effects of LEO (using bipolar electrocautery) versus gonadotrophin ovulation induction. This study followed up the participants ($n = 168$) of the largest RCT of LEO versus gonadotrophin therapy for up to 12 years. The long-term cumulative pregnancy rate (at least one pregnancy) after LEO was 86%, which was comparable to that of gonadotrophins (8). This high intrauterine pregnancy rate following LEO clearly demonstrated that postoperative adhesion formation seems to have little or no clinical significance.

Discussion

Laparoscopic electrocautery of the ovary has been widely accepted as the second-line treatment of choice for induction of ovulation in CC-resistant PCOS women in preference to gonadotrophin therapy. In addition to its proven efficacy, LEO offers several advantages over gonadotrophins, such as avoiding risks of multiple pregnancies and OHSS and reducing costs. However, critics say that LEO is an invasive procedure that requires general anesthetic and subjects the patient to risks, such as viscus injuries. Another major concern over LEO is the iatrogenic adhesion formation with a reported incidence of 30%–40%. However, as discussed above, the high long-term pregnancy rates with low ectopic pregnancy rates after LEO suggest that post-LEO adhesions have no clinical significance. Furthermore, adhesions can be largely minimized by avoiding thermal injury to the ovarian surface. Another risk associated with LEO is premature ovarian insufficiency (POI) possibly due to excessive destruction of the normal ovarian follicles or the inadvertent damage of the ovarian blood supply. Recent research has provided some evidence of a possible damage to ovarian reserve following LEO as determined by a postoperative fall in circulating anti-Müllerian hormone and rise in serum FSH concentration. However, these data should be interpreted with caution, given the limited reliability of these markers and the lack of any long term follow-up data. Furthermore, many long-term follow up studies have confirmed safety of LEO with no evidence of any premature ovarian failure. Excessive ovarian damage can be largely avoided by minimizing the amount of energy delivered, reducing the number of punctures, and avoiding the ovarian hilum.

Conclusion

In conclusion, LEO should be considered in women with CC-resistant PCOS as a safe and effective fertility treatment. It offers comparable live birth rates to gonadotrophin therapy with the added benefit of reducing the risks of multiple pregnancies and avoiding OHSS. Patients could expect 50%–60% pregnancy rates during 12 months following LEO. Monopolar and bipolar techniques seem to be equally effective with proven short- and long-term safety. The role of LEO before ART remains controversial. In addition to the short-term benefits of LEO, up to half of the patients undergoing this surgery will continue to benefit for several years.

TABLE 18.1

Level of Evidence of Statements

Statement	Level of Evidence
LEO is not superior to CC as a first-line treatment in anovulatory PCOS women.	1b
LEO and gonadotrophins are equally effective in inducing ovulation and generating pregnancies in CC-resistant PCOS women.	1a
LEO is associated with lower risks of multiple pregnancy compared to gonadotrophins.	1a
Four punctures (7–8 mm deep) per ovary with a power setting of 30–40 watts for 5 seconds per puncture seem to be the optimum dose of monopolar ovarian electrocautery.	2
Approximately, 50% of PCOS women continue to benefit from LEO for many years.	2
Both bipolar and monopolar techniques of LEO have proven long-term safety.	2

TABLE 18.2

Grade of Strength for Recommendations

Recommendation	Grade Strength
LEO cannot be recommended as a first-line treatment in anovulatory PCOS women.	A
Clomiphene citrate–resistant PCOS women should make an informed choice between LEO and gonadotrophin therapy, which are equally effective with possible advantages of LEO.	A
When using monopolar electrocautery, four punctures (7–8 mm deep) should be made into the anti-mesentric side of each ovary with a power setting of 30 watts for 5 seconds per puncture with minimal or no thermal damage to the ovarian surface.	B
LEO may be recommended in gonadotrophin-over-respondent PCOS women.	B

REFERENCES

1. Amer S, Li TC, Emarh M, Metwally M, Ledger WL. Randomized controlled trial comparing laparoscopic ovarian diathermy with clomifene citrate as a first line method of ovulation induction in women with polycystic ovarian syndrome. Hum Reprod. 2009; 24:219–25.
2. Farquhar C, Brown J, Marjoribanks J. Laparosocpic drilling by diathermie or laser for ovulation induction in anovulatory polycystic ovary syndrome. Cochrane Database Syst Rev. 2012; CD001122.
3. Bayram N, van Wely M, Kaaijk EM, Bossuyt PM, van der Veen F. Using an electrocautery strategy or recombinant follicle stimulating hormone to induce ovulation in polycystic ovary syndrome: Randomised controlled trial. BMJ. 2004; 328:192.
4. Nahuis MJ, Kose N, Bayram N, van Dessel HJ, Braat DD, Hamilton CJ et al. Long-term outcomes in women with polycystic ovary syndrome initially randomized to receive laparoscopic electrocautery of the ovaries or ovulation induction with gonadotrophins. Hum Reprod. 2011; 26:1899–904.
5. Amer S, Li TC, Cooke ID. A prospective dose finding study of the amount of energy required for laparoscopic ovarian diathermy in women with polycystic ovarian syndrome. Hum Reprod. 2003; 18:1693–8.
6. Amer SA, Li TC, Cooke ID. Laparoscopic ovarian diathermy in women with polycystic ovarian syndrome: A retrospective study on the influence of the amount of energy used on the outcome. Hum. Reprod. 2002; 17:1046–51.
7. Amer S, Li TC, Gopalan V, Ledger WL, Cooke ID. Long term follow up of patients with polycystic ovarian syndrome after laparoscopic ovarian drilling: Clinical outcome. Hum Reprod. 2002; 17:2035–42.
8. Nahuis MJ, Oude Lohuis EJ, Kose N, Bayram N, Hompes P, Oosterhuis GJ et al. Long-term follow-up of laparoscopic electrocautery of the ovaries versus ovulation induction with recombinant FSH in clomiphene citrate-resistant women with polycystic ovary syndrome: An economic evaluation. Hum Reprod. 2012; 27:3577–82.

19

Treatment of WHO 2: Gonadotropins and the Role of GnRH Agonists and Antagonists

Jean-Noël Hugues and Isabelle Cédrin-Durnerin

Introduction

Polycystic ovary syndrome (PCOS) is the most common form of WHO 2 anovulation, characterized by a normo-gonadotrophic and normo-estrogenic hormonal pattern. In women who failed to ovulate following clomiphene citrate (CC resistant) or to conceive following CC treatment (CC failure), gonadotropins are usually the next line of treatment. As polycystic ovaries are extremely sensitive to gonadotropins, ovulation induction with exogenous gonadotropins carries a high risk for multiple follicle recruitment, ovarian hyper-stimulation syndrome (OHSS) and multiple pregnancies.

The issue of how to prescribe gonadotropins was addressed many years ago. Although induction of ovulation using gonadotropin was first initiated in 1961, no guidelines of prescription were provided at that time. A major advance was the report by Brown of his clinical experience. Indeed, Brown proposed in 1978 the concept of a FSH threshold, emphasizing that the ovarian requirement for FSH operates in a very narrow range (1). The principle was to determine the individual dose of FSH leading to the development of the most sensitive follicle. As this threshold dose may hugely differ between individuals, he suggested a stepwise FSH increment by no more than 30% in agreement with the elevation of serum FSH during the early follicular phase. This observation allowed the development of the so-called "step-up protocols," which are now the gold standard in many centers. It was a major breakthrough to reduce the risk of overstimulation often associated with ovarian stimulation in patients with WHO 2 anovulation.

Overview of Existing Evidence

Step-Up Regimens

Step-up protocols are the most commonly used, at least for the first stimulation cycle. Indeed, it allows the assessment of the individual ovarian responsiveness to FSH by determining the dose required to induce the development of the most sensitive follicle of the cohort.

In the early 1980s, the use of conventional dose (150 IU/d) in conjunction with a rapid dose increment in absence of follicular growth was associated with high rates of cycle cancellation or multiple pregnancies due to multi-follicular development. Therefore, a subtle adjustment of both the starting dose and the dose increment was recommended in order to carefully achieve the FSH threshold for follicular growth. As soon as a selected follicle has emerged, the same dose is maintained up to the time of hCG administration. This principle of step-up administration of gonadotropins was applied with the low-dose and chronic low-dose protocols that proved to be safer than the conventional one. In nonobese patients, the recommended starting daily dose of FSH is 37.5 to 50 UI. A strict adhesion to a first step of 14 days was associated with a reduction in the risk of multi-follicular development. Adjustment in the dose every

5–7 days was justified because, due to the long FSH half-life, it took about 5 days to get a steady state of serum FSH. The increment at any stage of the stimulation should not exceed 50% in order to reduce the risk of over-response. In absence of pregnancy, treatment of the subsequent cycle generally begins at the threshold of response previously determined. Due to the possible cycle-to-cycle variability of the individual ovarian response, a close monitoring of each cycle is recommended. In absence of ovarian response to a daily dose of 225 IU or after 35–42 days of treatment, ovarian stimulation is usually cancelled.

Step-Down Regimen

An alternative was proposed to mimic physiology more closely. The step-down protocol aimed at administering an initial loading dose of gonadotropin to surpass the FSH threshold (2). Subsequently, when a follicle emerges from the cohort, the daily dose is reduced in order to close the FSH window. This regimen allowed a decrease in the duration of FSH administration but needs more experience and skill to avoid an ovarian hyper-response or a drop in follicular growth.

Efficacy and Safety of Different Regimens

There is no doubt that application of the low-dose and the chronic low-dose step-up regimens was associated with higher efficacy and safety than the conventional use of FSH. Using the chronic low-dose regimen (CLD), reported results showed a remarkably consistent rate of mono-ovulatory cycles of around 70% and an acceptable pregnancy rate of 20% per cycle. In addition, the risk of ovarian hyper-stimulation syndrome was significantly reduced and the rate of multiple pregnancies was <6% (3). Fair cumulative conception rates were reported (60% at 6 months).

Few studies have compared the efficacy and the safety of CLD step-up and step-down protocols in the first stimulation cycle. Even if the clinical characteristics of patients included in these studies were not comparable, the risk of over-response appeared to be high with the step-down regimen as a first-line therapy because the FSH threshold dose was not previously assessed. Therefore, it seemed safer to offer first a "dose-finding" CLD step-up induction cycle. In the next cycle, a step-down regimen can be applied with a starting dose 37.5 IU above the effective response dose individually determined. Using this approach, both protocols showed comparable ovulation and pregnancy rates with a low risk of multiple pregnancy and OHSS. Nevertheless, the small number of patients included in these studies and the heterogeneity between PCOS women limit the conclusion of these trials.

These data also show that a strict monitoring of ovarian stimulation is highly recommended. Both ultrasound assessment and hormonal determination during all cycles are useful at about a weekly interval to adjust the dose and prevent over-response. Criteria for cancellation due to an over-response should be discussed with couples before engaging gonadotropin treatment. During the last decade, a consensus has been reached to take into account the overall number of follicles >10 mm. In the youngest (≤32 years) women, stimulation should be cancelled and triggering of ovulation withholding in the presence of more than three follicles ≥14 mm associated with serum estradiol level above 1.000 pg/ml (3.671 pmol/L). Nevertheless, it seems relevant to adjust criteria for cycle cancellation to women's age and to the type and duration of infertility as well. The policy is clearly to prevent the risk of high-order multiple pregnancies.

These data emphasize the need to determine the individual effective starting dose and the risk of over-response by using a prediction model.

Predictive Factors for Success and Complications

The development of prediction models was initiated in the early 2000s to improve both efficacy and safety of ovulation-induction regimens. This approach was helpful for individualization of regimens and to inform patients about the risk of multiple pregnancies.

The choice of the optimal starting dose of FSH is critical for prevention of ovarian over-response (2). A prediction model was developed for the FSH response dose during the initial dose-finding treatment cycle, consisting of the following parameters: body mass index (BMI), cycle history, resistance to clomiphene citrate, free insulin-like growth factor I (IGF-I), and initial serum FSH concentrations. This model was validated in different WHO 2 ovulation induction groups stimulated with a low-dose protocol. It confirmed that BMI is the most relevant clinical parameter for the choice of the starting dose. More recently, it has been reported that, in women with PCOS, determination of serum AMH may be helpful in determining the starting FSH dose. Women with high AMH values should require a higher dose of FSH in agreement with the concept that AMH exerts a negative effect on ovarian FSH sensitivity. These new data deserve confirmation throughout additional prospective clinical trials.

Regarding the risk of multi-follicular development during FSH ovulation induction, it can be predicted by the degree of hyperandrogenism (total testosterone and androstenedione), the level of basal LH, and the antral follicular count (AFC). This confirms that the severity of PCOS phenotype is associated with a high risk of over-response due to the androgen-related increase in the number of follicles.

These predictive models have been externally validated. In addition, a retrospective analysis of first CLD cycles performed in more than 400 women with WHO 2 anovulation confirmed that normal BMI, AFC and FSH values in the upper part of the normal range are usually associated with successful ovulation induction with a low risk of cancellation for hypo- or hyper-response (4).

Finally, the main predictor of the chance for ongoing pregnancy was women's age. This is line with the results of a large multicenter study of 335 patients treated with strictly defined and monitored protocols. They showed that the three simple pretreatment parameters—(a) duration of infertility, (b) basal serum FSH concentration, and (c) the menstrual cycle status—were predictive of live birth after ovulation induction with gonadotropins in normogonadotropic anovulation.

Using these prediction models is the best way for clinicians to individualize regimens according to patients' characteristics and to counsel couples on their chance to achieve pregnancy with this therapy. The ultimate goal is to reduce the risk of high-order multiple pregnancies and OHSS.

Type of Gonadotropin Used

As women with WHO 2 anovulation display basal serum FSH and LH concentrations within the normal range and an adequate estrogenic impregnation, supplementation of these patients with FSH alone is usually recommended. It is even more evident for PCOS women whose basal serum LH concentration is elevated. Nevertheless, both FSH and human menopausal gonadotropins (hMG containing FSH and LH in a ratio 1/1) have been used with similar cycle outcome. The recent development of recombinant technologies allowed the production of FSH with a higher bioactivity as compared to urinary products. Indeed, pooled analysis of six clinical trials (5) reported a significantly shorter duration of treatment with rFSH compared with uFSH, and the weighted means for the total FSH dose were lower during treatment with rFSH. In addition, a significantly higher ovulation rate was observed after rFSH in comparison to urinary products, but this did not lead to a higher pregnancy rate. Finally, the availability of pens for administration of recombinant Follitropin alpha and beta make these products more convenient due to the ease of self-administration with less pain compared to conventional syringe and vials. Although recombinant products are more expensive than the urinary products, the cost-effectiveness of the two preparations does not seem to be quite different.

Role of GnRH Analogs

The interest of a concomitant administration of a GnRH agonist and gonadotropin to improve pregnancy rates in patients undergoing ovulation induction has not been firmly established. Additionally, combined therapy was associated with an increased risk of OHSS, and there are insufficient data to draw solid conclusions on miscarriage and multiple pregnancy rates. Therefore, the significantly higher hyperstimulation rate, the additional inconvenience, and cost of concomitant GnRH agonist administration, in the absence of documented increases in pregnancy success, do not justify the routine use of GnRH agonists during ovulation induction with gonadotropins in PCOS patients.

The question of whether LH suppression by a GnRH antagonist during gonadotropin-based ovulation induction is of benefit to women with PCOS has not yet been proven. One of the advantages could be to reduce the risk of premature progesterone levels that is not actually frequent during light ovarian stimulations (LOE 1a). The increased cost and the absence of improved pregnancy rate cannot justify, so far, the prescription of GnRH antagonist, at least when IUI has not been simultaneously scheduled.

Discussion

Ovulation induction with gonadotropins is still a challenging issue. Because most patients are highly sensitive to FSH and LH, the risk of over-response associated with OHSS and high-order multiple pregnancies is still a concern. Based on clinical experience, the development of step-up and step-down protocols did really improve both efficacy and safety of ovarian stimulation. That way, a large majority of anovulatory women can achieve a singleton pregnancy and the risk of over-response is dramatically reduced. Nevertheless, couples should be informed that ovarian stimulation is not always safe, and clinicians should strictly adhere to criteria for frequent monitoring and cycle cancellation. The use of prediction models was efficient to reduce the physical and psychological burden of ovarian stimulation that requires an intense ovarian response monitoring. However, further refinement is needed to better control safety and secure efficiency. Indeed, preventing all multiple pregnancies and OHSS is not possible at this time. The concomitant use of GnRH analogs does not improve cycle outcome.

Conclusions

WHO 2 anovulation is a common disorder in infertile women. Induction of ovulation with gonadotropins is usually a second-line therapy. Its effectiveness has been largely proven, but it requires experience and skill to get a singleton live birth, the ultimate goal of this therapy.

TABLE 19.1

Level of Evidence of Statements

Statement	Level of Evidence
In women with WHO 2 anovulation as the main cause of infertility, the use of step-up protocols significantly reduces the risk of multiple pregnancies.	1a
The starting dose of gonadotropins and the risk of over-response can be assessed by prediction models.	1a
A frequent monitoring every 5–7 days using ultrasound assessment and hormonal determination is able to prevent the risk of over-response.	1b
The safety of low-dose and chronic low-dose protocols is higher than the conventional one.	1b
Small FSH dose increments of 50% of the initial or previous FSH dose are less likely to result in excessive stimulation.	1b
When more than three growing follicles are observed on ultrasound in young women, the risk of multiple pregnancies is increased.	1b
The concomitant use of a GnRH agonist and gonadotropins does not improve pregnancy rates and is associated with an increased risk of OHSS.	1a
The introduction of GnRH antagonist during stimulation for WHO 2 anovulation is not absolutely required except in presence of premature progesterone elevation.	1b

TABLE 19.2

Grade of Strength for Recommendations

Recommendation	Grade Strength
Although sometimes difficult to achieve, the goal of gonadotropin treatment is to promote the growth and development of a single mature follicle.	A
The starting dose of gonadotropin needs to be adjusted according to the patient's BMI: 37.5 to 75 IU/day in non-obese women, 75 to 112.5 IU in obese women.	A
Adherence to a 14-day starting period at least for the first cycle is less likely to result in excessive stimulation.	A
The dose increments should not exceed 50% of the preceding dose.	A
After six ovulatory cycles using gonadotropins, strategy needs to be reconsidered with the couple.	B
Low-dose FSH protocols are effective in achieving ovulation in women with WHO 2 anovulation, but further refinement is needed to better control the safety of these regimens.	A
Intense ovarian response monitoring is required to reduce complications and secure efficiency.	A
Strict cycle cancellation criteria should be agreed upon with the patient before therapy is started.	A
Preventing all multiple pregnancies and OHSS is not possible at this time.	A

REFERENCES

1. Brown JB. Pituitary control of ovarian function–concepts derived from gonadotrophin therapy. Aust NZ J Obstet Gynaec. 1978; 18(1):47–54.
2. Van Santbrink EJP, Eijkemans MJ, Laven JSE, Fauser BCJM. Patient-tailored conventional ovulation algorithms in anovulatory infertility. Trends Endocrinol Metab. 2005; 16(8):381–9.
3. Homburg R, Howles CM. Low dose FSH therapy for anovulatory infertility associated with polycystic ovary syndrome: Rationale, reflections and refinements. Hum Reprod Update. 1999; 5(5):493–9.
4. Howles CM, Alam V, Tredway D, Homburg R, Warne DW. Factors related to successful ovulation induction in patients with WHO group II anovulatory infertility. Reprod BioMed Online. 2010; 20(2):182–90.
5. Nahuis M, van der Veen F, Oosterhuis J, Mol BW, Hompes P, van Wely M. Review of the safety, efficacy, costs and patient acceptability of recombinant follicle-stimulating hormone for injection in assisting ovulation induction in infertile women. Int J Women's Health. 2009; 9(1):205–11.

20

Treatment of WHO 2: Lifestyle Modifications

Walter Kuchenbecker, Helena J. Teede, and Lisa J. Moran

Introduction

Anovulation is the primary cause of subfertility in 15%–20% of women seeking fertility care. Normogonadotrophic, normoestrogenic anovulation (WHO 2) occurs commonly, and about 91% of women with WHO 2 anovulation fit the broader diagnostic criteria of polycystic ovary syndrome (PCOS) (1). PCOS occurs in up to 6%–18% of reproductive-age women, depending on the population studied. PCOS accounts for 70%–90% of all ovulatory disorders (2). Women are diagnosed as PCOS according to the Rotterdam consensus diagnostic criteria if two of the following criteria are identified: anovulation, clinical or biochemical hyperandrogenemia, or polycystic ovary morphology on ultrasound and after other endocrine causes of anovulation are excluded (2). The clinical manifestation of PCOS is variable due to the heterogeneity of PCOS being influenced by factors, including ethnicity, body weight, and body fat distribution. Women with PCOS may have a propensity to gain weight. Although the literature is variable, overweight and obesity are common in PCOS (pooled estimated prevalence of 61%, 95% CI 54–68), according to the WHO criteria.

Mechanisms of Anovulation

The pathophysiology of PCOS remains unclear but is most likely based on a multifactorial origin with a combination of genetic and environmental factors. Considerable evidence indicates that insulin resistance and the resulting hyperinsulinemia is the etiologic feature in 95% of obese and 75% of lean women with PCOS, and hyperandrogenemia can be detected in 60%–80% of women with PCOS (3).

Insulin resistance contributes to lower sex hormone binding globulin (SHBG) concentrations and, consequently, higher free androgen levels. High androgen levels directly influence intra-ovarian steroidogenesis, which leads to arrest of follicle growth and anovulation.

Obesity, in particular abdominal and visceral obesity, contributes to insulin resistance and a subsequent decrease in SHBG and increase in hyperandrogenemia. Excess weight therefore increases the risk of developing PCOS and overweight or obesity contributes to a more severe phenotype of PCOS with regards to the reproductive, psychological, and metabolic consequences.

Adipose tissue can store androgens, convert androgen precursors to active androgens, and secrete various peptides, collectively called adipocytokines. Increasing BMI can contribute to dysfunctional adipose tissue with increased secretion of pro-inflammatory adipocytokines and decreased secretion of adiponectin, an insulin-sensitizing adipocytokine. Altered regulation of adipocytokines, including leptin and adiponectin, may contribute to anovulation through effects on hypothalamic function, insulin resistance, or the ovary.

This chapter will aim to discuss lifestyle modification as a measure to achieve weight loss and resumption of ovulation in women with WHO 2 anovulation.

Lifestyle Modification

The optimal lifestyle modification program for achieving weight loss consists of dietary intervention and exercise in combination with behavior modification. The existing literature mainly addresses lifestyle modification in at-risk groups (including those at an elevated risk of developing DM2 or cardiovascular disease) of the general population and in anovulatory women with PCOS, but these findings can also be extrapolated to the group of non-PCOS women with WHO 2 anovulation.

Weight Loss and Prevention of Weight Gain (3)

In populations at risk for DM2, many randomized controlled trials (RCTs) report that lifestyle modification leads to weight loss, improvement in insulin sensitivity, decreased prevalence of DM2, and decreased risk factors for cardiovascular disease when compared to placebo or insulin-sensitizing drugs. Long-term weight loss and weight maintenance should be managed by long-term support in maintaining a healthy diet and increased exercise in combination with behavior modification. Lifestyle modification during pregnancy and limiting weight gain during pregnancy and modest preconception weight loss when women are overweight or obese can also contribute to improved fertility or a decrease in obesity-related pregnancy complications (LOE 1a) (4).

Many small and uncontrolled trials indicate that weight loss achieved through lifestyle modification in overweight/obese women with or without PCOS leads to loss of abdominal fat, improvement in insulin sensitivity, and decrease in hyperandrogenemia.

In overweight/obese women with PCOS, a modest weight loss of 5%–10% of total body weight leads to improvement of menstrual cyclicity and resumption of ovulation in up to 60% of these women. Small, uncontrolled trials have shown that loss of visceral fat and improvement in insulin resistance is required for resumption of ovulation in overweight/obese women with PCOS. One high-quality systematic review that assessed six RCTs showed that lifestyle modification in women with PCOS improves markers of insulin resistance and weight and central fat compared to minimal treatment or usual care (LOE 1a). There were minimal data available on clinical reproductive outcomes, such as resumption of ovulation or conception rates.

Based on general population data and emerging data in PCOS, lifestyle modification for weight loss in overweight/obese women with WHO 2 anovulation and prevention of weight gain in lean women should be recommended for improving general health, well-being, and reproductive outcomes (Table 20.2).

Diet and Macronutrient Composition (3)

Dietary interventions should be tailored to the personal preferences of each individual woman and should aim to achieve a calorie reduction of 600 kcal/d. There is considerable interest in the concept that weight loss and other favorable health outcomes can be influenced by changing the macronutrient composition (fat, carbohydrate, or protein content) of a diet. The effect of the macronutrient composition of the dietary intervention during lifestyle modification on weight loss in the general population has been assessed by many RCTs and systematic reviews. The findings of these studies are not conclusive and differ in terms of the amount of weight loss achieved during lifestyle modification, the intensity and duration of the lifestyle intervention, and the follow-up period.

Five RCTs compared the macronutrient composition of dietary intervention in women with PCOS comprising low-carbohydrate, low-glycemic index, monounsaturated fatty acid enriched, high-protein, carbohydrate-counting, fat-counting, or conventional healthy diets.

In comparison to a conventional healthy diet, there were no differences in the majority of anthropometric and fertility (menstrual regularity, ovulation, or pregnancy) outcomes. Specifically with regards to clinical reproductive outcomes, one study reported increased menstrual regularity for 95% of women after a low glycemic index ad libitum weight-loss diet compared with 63% of women following a standard healthy ad libitum weight-loss diet.

Evidence-based guidelines recommend that lifestyle modification regimens should incorporate a dietary intake consistent with popular dietary guideline recommendations as opposed to a modified macronutrient composition. This can be followed for weight maintenance, prevention of weight gain in lean women with PCOS, or as a moderately calorie-restricted approach for achieving weight loss in overweight or obese women with PCOS.

Exercise (3)

Increased aerobic exercise improves cardiopulmonary function and insulin sensitivity and has a favorable effect on general well-being and health-related quality of life (QOL). Moderate aerobic exercise is defined as an intensity between 50% and 80% of maximum oxygen consumption or 60%–90% of maximal heart rate. Studies in high-risk subjects reveal that moderate exercise of at least three to five times per week reduces DM2 risk and improves cardiovascular risk profile.

Exercise compared to no exercise or different exercises: In PCOS, five RCTs comparing exercise to no exercise showed some improvement in markers of insulin resistance.

However, the effect on other outcomes, such as BMI, waist-hip ratio, and blood pressure, were inconsistent, and these studies did not assess resumption of ovulation. Exercise also consists of aerobic or resistance exercise with specific health benefits occurring with both types of training. Resistance exercise alone or combined with aerobic exercise improves health outcomes in high-risk groups when compared to no exercise. Specifically in PCOS, RCTs comparing aerobic exercise to combined aerobic and resistance exercise showed no differences in fat mass, fat-free mass, and QOL.

Exercise with or without dietary intervention: A low-quality non-RCT with a high risk of bias compared a structured exercise program (SET) to a high protein diet (800 kcal deficit per day) in obese women (BMI ≥33.1 kg/m^2) with PCOS. The SET group showed greater improvement in menstrual frequency ($P = 0.04$) and ovulation rates ($P = 0.03$) compared to the diet group. SET also showed more improvement in markers of insulin sensitivity, and the diet intervention achieved greater changes in weight and BMI for participants who ovulated ($P < 0.05$).

A randomized, parallel study of 94 overweight and obese women with PCOS (BMI 36.1 ± 4.8 kg/m^2) undergoing a 20-week lifestyle intervention program assessed the effects of aerobic and aerobic-resistance exercise combined with an energy-restricted high protein diet (1195–1434 kcal/d) on metabolic risk factors and reproductive function. There was no difference in weight loss between the three groups, but aerobic (DA) and aerobic-resistance (DC) exercise combined with an energy-restricted high-protein diet showed more decease in fat mass (3 kg) with less decrease of fat-free mass compared to the dietary intervention alone (DO) ($P ≤ 0.03$). With regards to reproductive outcomes, in 53 women with menstrual irregularities, there were no differences in menstrual cyclicity improvements between the three groups, but women in the DA group had a greater number of ovulatory cycles than in the DO group (DO 1.33 ± 1.63, DA 3.10 ± 1.97; $P = 0.04$).

In another RCT, 57 overweight/obese PCOS women were randomized to 4 months of DO, exercise only (EO), or combined diet and exercise (DE). Weight loss was more pronounced in the DO (–6%) and DE (–5%) group compared to the EO (–3%) group.

Lean body mass was preserved in the exercise groups (DE and EO). The menstrual pattern improved significantly in 69% of women, and ovulation was confirmed in 34% of women with no differences between the groups (5).

Evidence-based guidelines recommend that lifestyle modification for weight loss in overweight/obese women with WHO 2 anovulation should combine dietary intervention (reduced calorie intake) and exercise as a first-line therapy (LOE 1a). Exercise of at least 150 minutes per week should be recommended of which 90 minutes should entail moderate- to high-intensity exercise (60%–90% of maximum heart rate).

Behavior Modification (3)

Behavior modification is essential to achieve maximal compliance and adherence to lifestyle modification and to limit attrition. Models used to enhance improvements in patients behavior entail important elements, such as encouraging self-monitoring, setting goals, enhancing self-efficacy, increasing knowledge, and providing feedback.

In the general population, research indicates that the application of behavior change techniques (motivational interviewing, stages of change model, and others) and increasing the frequency, intensity, and duration of contact with a health professional results in greater weight loss. Engaging the spouse, family, or a personal friend for social support during lifestyle modification also enhances adherence and compliance. Tailoring lifestyle modification to the personal circumstances and preferences of the patient is advisable. A wide range of health care providers, including doctors, nurses, dietitians, nutritionists, psychologists, and exercise specialists, can provide and deliver the necessary care to assist the patient in achieving changes in behavior in an individual, group, or mixed setting.

Seven RCTs comparing different dietary delivery methods during lifestyle modification in women with PCOS reported no differences in weight loss between the interventions. All studies consistently involved dietitian consultation with some differences present in the frequency and intensity of monitoring across the studies.

Evidence-based guidelines recommend that lifestyle modification for weight loss in overweight/obese women and prevention of weight gain in lean women with WHO 2 anovulation should entail face-to-face dietary advice and education on healthy food choices and exercise accompanied by behavior change techniques, personal guidance, and support (LOE 1a). Lifestyle modification is the joint responsibility of all health care professionals who are involved in the care of women with WHO 2 anovulation.

Weight management refers not only to achieving modest weight loss, but also to maintaining this weight loss long term. Long-term weight maintenance is very difficult for all individuals. Many women with WHO 2 anovulation who are overweight or obese are therefore at risk of regaining weight over time after initial weight loss. Long-term low-intensity support for behavior modification strategies aimed at preventing relapse and maintaining positive changes in exercise and dietary intake have been shown to limit weight gain over time.

In adult women with PCOS and a BMI ≥35 kg/m^2 who remain infertile despite attempting to achieve weight loss through an intensive lifestyle modification program for a minimum of 6 months and/or pharmacological therapy, bariatric surgery could be considered a second-line therapy. Bariatric surgery should only be performed in a multidisciplinary setting in order to optimize outcomes and limit complications. Patients should be counseled to avoid conception during the period of rapid weight loss after bariatric surgery due to the increased risk of small for gestational-age newborns and women should only aim to conceive after 12–18 months when maximal weight loss is achieved (3).

Conclusion

Weight loss in overweight/obese women with WHO 2 anovulation leads to improvement in insulin sensitivity and decreases in hyperandrogenemia, which contribute to resumption of ovulation.

Lifestyle modification for weight loss and resumption of ovulation in overweight/obese women and prevention of weight gain in lean women with WHO 2 anovulation should entail dietary intervention (reduced calorie intake of 600 kcal/d) and exercise in combination with behavior modification as a first-line therapy (LOE 1a).

TABLE 20.1

Level of Evidence of Statements

Statement	Level of Evidence
Modest weight loss achieved by lifestyle modification in overweight/obese women with WHO 2 anovulation contributes to resumption of ovulation.	2a
Limiting weight gain in women who are overweight or obese by means of lifestyle modification during pregnancy improves obstetric outcomes.	1a
Lifestyle modification for weight loss should include a healthy diet (reduced calorie intake) and increased exercise in combination with behavior modification.	1a

TABLE 20.2

Grade of Strength for Recommendations

Recommendation	Grade Strength
Lifestyle modification targeting weight loss in overweight/obese women with WHO 2 anovulation and prevention of weight gain in lean women should be recommended for improving general health and well-being.	B
Preconception weight loss in overweight/obese women and limiting weight gain during pregnancy should be advised with the aim to decrease obesity-related pregnancy complications.	C
Lifestyle modification targeting weight loss in overweight/obese women with WHO 2 anovulation and prevention of weight gain in lean women should entail the combination of reduced calorie intake and increased exercise in combination with behavior modification.	C
Lifestyle modification for weight loss in overweight/obese women with WHO 2 anovulation and prevention of weight gain in lean women should entail face-to-face dietary advice and education on healthy food choices (irrespective of macronutrient composition) and instructions on increased exercise accompanied by behavior change techniques, personal guidance, and support.	D

REFERENCES

1. ESHRE Capri Workshop Group. Health and fertility in World Health Organization group 2 anovulatory women. Hum Reprod Update. 2012; 18(5):586–99.
2. Legro RS, Arslanian SA, Ehrmann DA et al. Diagnosis and treatment of polycystic ovary syndrome: An Endocrine Society clinical practice guideline. J Clin Endocrinol Metab. 2013; 98(12):4565–92.
3. Teede HJ, Misso ML, Deeks AA et al. Assessment and management of polycystic ovary syndrome: Summary of an evidence-based guideline. Med J Aust. 2011; 195(6):S65–112.
4. NICE guidelines: Weight management before, during and after pregnancy. 2010; PH27.
5. Nybacka A, Carlstrom K, Stahle A, Nyren S, Hellstrom PM, Hirschberg AL. Randomized comparison of the influence of dietary management and/or physical exercise on ovarian function and metabolic parameters in overweight women with polycystic ovary syndrome. Fertil Steril. 2011; 96(6):1508–13.

21

Treatment of WHO 3

Annelien C. de Kat, Scott M. Nelson, and Frank J. M. Broekmans

Introduction

Primary ovarian insufficiency (POI), also known as World Health Organization (WHO) type 3 amenorrhea, is defined by the existence of permanent ovarian insufficiency before the age of 40 and occurs in approximately 1% of the female population (1). It is the result of the accelerated decline of ovarian function, leading to hypergonadotropic hypogonadism. Ovarian insufficiency is clinically expressed by the combination of amenorrhea for a period of at least 6 months and elevated follicle-stimulating hormone (FSH) levels (>40 IU/l) (2,3). Further characteristics accompanying this condition are infertility and estrogen deficiency signs (4). There are several causes that can contribute to POI, of which idiopathic cases constitute the largest group (1). In addition, POI can be caused by genetic (such as Turner syndrome), autoimmune, environmental, or iatrogenic factors (5,6). For women with POI, although ovarian function is insufficient to ensure a monthly ovulatory cycle, there is still a small possibility of a spontaneous pregnancy occurring, with studies reporting rates varying from 2.5% to a maximum of 10% (1,7,8). This indicates that complete depletion of the follicle pool may not always be present. Therefore, attention has been given to applying ovarian stimulation to this group of patients in the hope of utilizing the last available follicular reserve and enabling the occurrence of ovulation.

It needs to be recognized however that folliculogenesis is a process that can be manipulated externally only to a limited extent. The continuous transition of follicles from the primordial pool and the subsequent development toward antral stages has classically been considered a process steered primarily by genetic, paracrine, and autocrine factors although the exact interplay of these factors remains to be elucidated. As such, it does not allow much room for manipulation from exogenous endocrine, immunologic, or metabolic factors with the exception of effects at the vascular or cytotoxic level, such as uterine artery embolization, ovarian surgery, or chemotherapy. Rather, it is the later cyclic phase of folliculogenesis that can be manipulated by endogenous signals from the pituitary–ovarian axis or by exogenous FSH and LH. However, depletion of the initial stages of the follicular development pathway will restrict the probability of successful induction of ovulation, and if this pool is (temporarily, but often permanently) absent, the chances of success may be considered futile.

This chapter will discuss evidence-based options for increasing the chances of natural conception through ovulation induction in patients with primary ovarian insufficiency. In addition, potential complications associated with subsequent pregnancy, including after oocyte donation, will be discussed.

Methods for Ovulation Induction

Pituitary Suppression

In the past 30 years, studies have sought to investigate whether pituitary suppression, be it through estrogen replacement or with an agonist of gonadotropin-releasing hormone (GnRH), contributes to a better outcome of ovulation induction in patients with primary ovarian insufficiency. It has been hypothesized that high levels of endogenous FSH in women with POI occupy FSH receptors, rendering them inaccessible for exogenous FSH for ovarian stimulation (9). Thus, lowering endogenous gonadotropins by pituitary suppression could possibly enable stimulation of otherwise resistant ovaries (9).

See Table 21.3 for a summary of clinical studies performed with regard to this method of ovulation induction in patients with WHO type 3 anovulation. A recent case report (10) described an ongoing pregnancy resulting from suppression with a GnRH agonist and estrogen therapy, followed by ovulation induction with exogenous gonadotropins (and luteal support with human chorionic gonadotropin [hCG]). In a crossover trial (11), patients with a normal karyotype POI received a daily dose of 300 µg of desrorelin, a GnRH receptor agonist, followed or preceded by a placebo phase. Estrogen replacement therapy

TABLE 21.3

Summary of Clinical Research Regarding Pituitary Suppression for Ovulation Induction in Patients with WHO Type 3 Anovulation

Author Name	Design	Patients	Treatment Regimen	Results
Nelson et al., 1992	CT	<40 years old, ≥4 months amenorrhea, serum FSH >40 IU/L on at least two occasions $N = 23$	300 µg deslorelin SC/day versus placebo SC/day + 2 mg oral micronized estrogen daily during both phases	13% ovulation after deslorelin; 9% ovulation after placebo ($p > 0.05$)
Van Kasteren et al., 1995	RCT	≤38 years old, secondary amenorrhea, FSH >40 IU/L on at least two occasions $N = 30$ ($n = 15$ per arm)	1 mg intranasal buserelin acetate daily versus placebo for 4 weeks + stimulation with 150 IU FSH daily until maximum 450 IU/day	20% ovulation with buserelin; 0/15 0% ovulation with placebo ($p > 0.05$)
Buckler et al., 1993	PT	≤36 years old, secondary amenorrhea, FSH >40 IU/L on at least two occasions, serum E2 <100 pmol/L $N = 8$	30 µg EE + 150 µg levonorgestrel daily for 12 weeks	No ovulation
Anasti et al., 1994	CT	<40 years old, ≥4 months amenorrhea, FSH >40 IU/L on at least two occasions $N = 46$	2 mg oral E_2 daily + 5 mg medroxyprogesterone acetate daily (HRT) versus 400 mg danazol daily	9% ovulatory progesterone level after HRT; 17% after danazol ($p > 0.05$)
Taylor et al., 1996	CT	<40 years old, ≥2 months amenorrhea, FSH >40 IU/L on at least two occasions $N = 32$	2 mg oral E_2 daily versus no treatment	42% ovulation during estrogen; 39% ovulation during no treatment ($p > 0.05$)
Tartagni et al., 2007	RCT	<40 years old, ≥6 months amenorrhea, FSH >40 IU/L and E_2 ≤25 pg/ml on at least two occasions $N = 50$ ($n = 25$ per arm)	0.05 mg EE 3× daily versus placebo + 200 IU r-βFSH	32% ovulation with EE; 0% ovulation with placebo ($p < 0.005$)
Check et al., 1990	PT	≤47 years old, ≥12 months amenorrhea, FSH and LH >35 IU/L $N = 100$	50–70 µg EE daily + hMG 150–375 IU/day	19% ovulation overall; 2.2% viable pregnancy per cycle
Surrey and Cedars, 1989	RCT	>12 months amenorrhea, FSH >40 IU/L $N = 14$	2.5 mg E_2 + hMG (A) 2.5 mg E_2 + hMG and 50 µg EE (B) 100 µg GnRH-a histrelin + hMG (C)	1/6 (17%) ovulation in group C, no ovulation in groups A and B

Note: CT = crossover trial; EE = ethinylestradiol; HRT = hormone replacement therapy; PT = prospective trial; RCT = randomized controlled trial.

was taken concomitantly. Ovulation was detected in 5 out of 23 women (22%), but the addition of des-rorelin was not found to increase the chance of ovulation (11). In 30 women with POI, suppression with buserelin, another GnRH agonist, was compared to placebo with subsequent stimulation with 10,000 IU hCG and 150 IU FSH with increasing doses to 450 IU daily (12). Luteal support was provided by 5000 IU hCG administration every 72 hours. There was no statistical difference between the incidence of ovu-lation in the treatment and placebo groups although ovulation did occur in three cases in the treatment group compared to none in the placebo group (12).

Estrogen replacement therapy is another method of pituitary suppression. In a study with eight women with POI (13), pituitary suppression with oral contraceptives did not lead to subsequent fol-licular growth or ovulation. The effect of danazol (a sex-steroid derivative) in comparison to estrogen–progestin treatment on ovarian and ovulatory function was studied in a crossover trial (14), showing no statistical differences in ovulation rate. An ovulation occurred in 21% of all included 52 patients (14). Another crossover trial did not find a difference in ovulation or pregnancy rate after estradiol treatment compared to no treatment although high rates of ovulation were reported in both groups (46% in the treatment group compared to 39% in the control group) (15). In a randomized trial with 50 patients, women with POI received ethinyl-estradiol or placebo before receiving 200 IU/day recombinant FSH for ovulation induction (16). The women who received estrogen treatment had a significantly higher ovulation rate (32% versus 0%) following ovulation induction, resulting in pregnancy in half of these cases (4/8) (16).

In a prospective cohort of 100 women with hypergonadotropic amenorrhea (17), gonadotropic sup-pression was reached through 50 µg ethinyl-estradiol daily, increasing the dose to 70 µg in a select group of patients with insufficient pituitary suppression. Subsequent induction using human menopausal gonadotropins (hMG) 150–375 IU/day was studied. Ovulation occurred in 19% of all induction cycles, and the viable pregnancy rate per cycle was 2.2% (17). A randomized trial was conducted in a total of 14 patients with POI (18), in which three treatment regimens were investigated: estrogen-induced sup-pression followed by stimulation with hMG; estrogen-induced suppression followed by hMG stimulation with concomitant estrogen therapy; and GnRH-agonist induced gonadotropin suppression followed by hMG stimulation. Ovulation occurred in a single patient in the latter group, and no pregnancies were reported (18).

All presented studies, with one exception (17), included patients younger than 40 years old with a history of amenorrhea and/or hypogonadism and FSH determined at two separate time points in a post-menopausal range (>35 mIU/ml). However, the duration of amenorrhea as a criterion for POI diagnosis was not always defined or even differed between studies, ranging from 4 months to >1 year. This dif-ference in applied diagnostic criteria could potentially impact the results and their interpretation. The duration of amenorrhea may have been associated with the degree of the remainder of ovarian reserve, expressed by the permanency level in the number of antral follicles responsive to exogenous FSH or lack thereof, thus greatly influencing the prognosis of ovulation induction.

In summary, pituitary suppression with a GnRH agonist does not seem to ameliorate the outcome of ovulation induction in patients with primary ovarian insufficiency (LOE 1b). Results concerning estro-gen replacement therapy are less consistent (LOE 1b). Ovulation rates after ovulation induction vary strongly in patients with POI but have been described to reach up to 42% (LOE 1b). Meta-analysis of the currently available data is not possible due to heterogeneity of the conducted trials (19). Differing diag-nostic criteria, use of different treatment protocols, and small sample sizes further limit comparability of results.

Corticosteroid Treatment

For some patients with idiopathic POI, an autoimmune pathophysiology has been suggested (7). Consequently, studies have assessed whether pretreatment with corticosteroids enhances the ovar-ian response to ovulation induction. See Table 21.4 for a summary of concerning studies. One trial comparing dexamethasone to placebo before treatment with 300 IU hMG was discontinued early due to no ovulation occurring in either the treatment or placebo group (20). In a more recent trial (21),

TABLE 21.4

Summary of Clinical Research Regarding Immunosuppressant Intervention for Ovulation Induction in Patients with WHO Type 3 Anovulation

Author Name	Design	Patients	Treatment Regimen	Results
Van Kasteren et al., 1999	RCT	≥4 months amenorrhea, FSH >40 IU/L N = 36	9 mg/day dexamethasone versus placebo + 300 IU hMG/day	No ovulation
Badawy et al., 2007	RCT	N = 58	6 mg/day dexamethasone versus placebo + 3.75 mg/day GnRH-a triptorelin + 300 IU/day hMG	20.7% ovulation with dexamethasone, 0% with placebo ($p < 0.05$)
Corenblum et al., 1993	PT	N = 11	25 mg 4×/day prednisone	2/11 (18%) ovulation leading to two viable pregnancies

Note: PT = prospective trial; RCT = randomized controlled trial.

patients were given a GnRH agonist and then randomized to gonadotropin therapy with dexamethasone or gonadotropin therapy with placebo. A 20.7% (6/29) ovulation rate was demonstrated in the dexamethasone group compared with 10.7% (3/29) in the placebo group, which reached statistical significance (21). In an uncontrolled group of 11 women receiving prednisone, an ovulation rate of 18% was found (22).

Thus, in patients with idiopathic POI, adding dexamethasone to a GnRH agonist may increase the likelihood of ovulation after ovulation induction compared to a GnRH agonist alone although further evidence is required (LOE 1b). There is additionally insufficient evidence to conclude whether corticosteroid treatment can increase the chance of spontaneous ovulation and subsequent pregnancy (LOE 1b).

Further Methods of Assisted Conception

In addition to the methods described, a number of adjuvant and alternative strategies have been examined in patients with WHO type 3 anovulation to facilitate conception.

Androgen Intervention

Dehydroepiandrosterone (DHEA) is a precursor of gonadal steroid hormones and consequently plays a role in follicular steroidogenesis. It has additionally been suggested to potentiate the effect of gonadotropins on follicle development, making it potentially beneficial for achieving the development of the few potentially remaining follicles in patients with POI. Treatment with DHEA did not improve markers of ovarian reserve or ovulation rate in patients with idiopathic POI in a randomized placebo-controlled trial (23) although the opposite was argued based on several case reports (24). There are currently no results of trials comparing DHEA treatment to placebo with subsequent ovulation induction.

Fertility Preservation

In the event of suspected or predicted accelerated ovarian decline, it may be possible to cryopreserve oocytes, embryos, or ovarian tissue before the complete depletion of the follicle pool. These techniques have, to date, primarily been used in females undergoing treatment for malignant disease with varying pregnancy rates (25), but their applicability to natural fertility decline have additionally been suggested (25). The process of successful fertility preservation has additionally been described in adolescents or women with Turner syndrome. With a greater role for ovarian reserve testing, women at risk for POI may be identified in an earlier stage, thus potentially increasing their options of achieving pregnancy. Initial research is required, however, to validate this technique for this specific group of patients. Animal studies suggest that transplantation of heterologous reproductive tissue may be possible, which would create another opportunity for women with POI, but this awaits further substantiation in human studies.

Oocyte Donation

Oocyte donation with an ongoing pregnancy as a result in a patient with POI was first described in a case report in 1984 (26). This method of conception is currently one of the most frequently used for patients with POI. Pregnancy rates resulting from oocyte donation are comparable, and sometimes superior, to those with other assisted reproduction techniques with rates varying from 20.5% to 58% (27,28). However, offspring from pregnancies following oocyte donation have an approximately 60% greater chance of being born prematurely and with a lower birth weight (27). In addition, maternal pregnancy complications are increased in pregnancies resulting from oocyte donation; increased risks of pregnancy-induced hypertension (31% versus 14%) (29), preeclampsia (17% versus 5%–10%) (28), placental abruption (1% absolute risk) (30), and cesarean section (75% absolute risk) (30–32). The latter results should be interpreted with maternal age as an important confounder in mind. Indeed, a study comparing obstetrical complications of oocyte donation-derived pregnancy in women with POI and women aged above 40 found the complication rate to be significantly higher in the older maternal age group (33). Nonetheless, taking into account the existing risk of obstetrical complications with the addition of the increasing risk of cardiovascular morbidity related to age at menopause (34), patients with POI and a pregnancy following oocyte donation should be considered as high risk. A more extreme risk can become manifest in pregnancy of women with Turner syndrome after oocyte donation due to preexisting cardiac malformations and cardiovascular sequelae associated with this syndrome (35). These considerations should be included in the counseling of women with POI for oocyte donation.

In conclusion, oocyte donation results in definitively higher pregnancy rates than ovulation induction in patients with POI (LOE 3). Pregnancies following oocyte donation are associated with an increased risk of perinatal and maternal complications (LOE 3). There is insufficient evidence to attribute a beneficial effect of androgen precursors on follicle development in the case of ovarian depletion (LOE 1b). Fertility preservation may be considered given the increasing possibility of early detection or prediction of POI (LOE 4).

Conclusion

Patients with POI have a small chance of conceiving spontaneously, making the usage of assisted reproduction techniques an important aspect of achieving pregnancy in this group of women. Studies concerning ovulation induction in these patients are scarce and quite heterogeneous. Another important limitation for the comparability of currently available literature is the use of different stimulation protocols and varying doses and combinations of treatment regimens. The interpretation of results is furthermore impeded due to small sample sizes, leading to underpowered studies. Undergoing treatment protocols for ovulation induction furthermore led to a significantly increased psychological burden in patients with POI (36), warranting a cautionary note in the implementation of treatment.

With the limited data available, it can be concluded that GnRH suppression does not increase ovulation rates. Moreover, currently there are no data indicating that adding DHEA does improve ovulation induction outcome. Inconsistent results are available regarding the use of estrogen replacement therapy in the regimen of ovulation induction, warranting further research. The same holds true for the role of corticosteroid administration in ovulation induction. It is wise to include a critical note, however, as the failure of ovulation induction is inherent to the physiologic state of primary ovarian insufficiency. Due to the limited effect of ovulation induction in patients with POI, oocyte donation is a more commonly used and reliable method for establishing pregnancy. When counseling for the latter option, increased risk of perinatal and maternal obstetric complications should be considered.

TABLE 21.1

Level of Evidence of Statements

Statement	Level of Evidence
Ovulation rates can reach up to 42% following ovulation induction.	1b
GnRH agonist pretreatment does not improve the results of ovulation induction.	1b
Estrogen therapy increased ovulation rate in a randomized trial, but this result is contradicted by smaller studies with a lower evidence level.	1b
Corticosteroid treatment may improve ovulation or pregnancy rates, but further research is required to substantiate this conclusion.	1b
Dehydroepiandrosterone does not improve the chances of ovulation or endocrine conditions in the ovary.	1b
Oocyte donation is more effective than ovulation induction for achieving pregnancy, but pregnancies following ovulation induction are more at risk for complications.	3

TABLE 21.2

Grade of Strength for Recommendations

Recommendation	Grade Strength
Patients with POI should be informed about the low probability of achieving pregnancy spontaneously or through ovulation induction.	B
When opting for ovulation induction, treatment schemes should be individualized due to lacking and contradicting existing evidence.	B
When considering oocyte donation, patients should be counseled about the increased risk of pregnancy complications.	C

REFERENCES

1. Coulam CB, Adamson SC, Annegers JF. Incidence of premature ovarian failure. Obstet Gynecol. 1986; 67(4):604–6.
2. Conway GS. Premature ovarian failure. Br Med Bull. 2000; 56(3):643–9.
3. Rebar RW, Connolly HV. Clinical features of young women with hypergonadotropic amenorrhea. Fertil Steril. 1990; 53(5):804–10.
4. Kalantaridou SN, Davis SR, Nelson LM. Premature ovarian failure. Endocrinol Metabol Clin North Am. 1998; 27(4):989–1006.
5. Goswami D, Conway GS. Premature ovarian failure. Hum Reprod Update. 2005; 11(4):391–410. dmi012 [pii]
6. Nelson LM. Clinical practice. primary ovarian insufficiency. N Engl J Med. 2009; 360(6):606–14. doi:10.1056/NEJMcp0808697
7. van Kasteren YM, Schoemaker J. Premature ovarian failure: A systematic review on therapeutic interventions to restore ovarian function and achieve pregnancy. Hum Reprod Update. 1999; 5(5):483–92.
8. Sauer MV. Spontaneous pregnancy in women awaiting oocyte donation. J Reprod Med. 1995; 40(9):630–2.
9. Hoek A, Schoemaker J, Drexhage HA. Premature ovarian failure and ovarian autoimmunity. Endocr Rev. 1997; 18(1):107–34. doi:10.1210/edrv.18.1.0291
10. Tsuji I, Ami K, Fujinami N. Pregnancy following ovarian induction in a patient with premature ovarian failure and undetectable serum anti-Mullerian hormone. J Obstet Gynaecol Res. 2013; 39(5):1070–2. doi:10.1111/j.1447-0756.2012.02068
11. Nelson LM, Kimzey LM, White BJ, Merriam GR. Gonadotropin suppression for the treatment of karyotypically normal spontaneous premature ovarian failure: A controlled trial. Fertil Steril. 1992; 57(1):50–5.
12. van Kasteren YM, Hoek A, Schoemaker J. Ovulation induction in premature ovarian failure: A placebo-controlled randomized trial combining pituitary suppression with gonadotropin stimulation. Fertil Steril. 1995; 64(2):273–8.

13. Buckler HM, Healy DL, Burger HG. Does gonadotropin suppression result in follicular development in premature ovarian failure? Gynecol Endocrinol. 1993; 7(2):123–8.
14. Anasti JN, Kimzey LM, Defensor RA, White B, Nelson LM. A controlled study of danazol for the treatment of karyotypically normal spontaneous premature ovarian failure. Fertil Steril. 1994; 62(4):726–30.
15. Taylor AE, Adams JM, Mulder JE, Martin KA, Sluss PM, Crowley WF Jr. A randomized, controlled trial of estradiol replacement therapy in women with hypergonadotropic amenorrhea. J Clin Endocrinol Metab. 1996; 81(10):3615–21. doi:10.1210/jcem.81.10.8855811
16. Tartagni M, Cicinelli E, De Pergola G, De Salvia MA, Lavopa C, Loverro G. Effects of pretreatment with estrogens on ovarian stimulation with gonadotropins in women with premature ovarian failure: A randomized, placebo-controlled trial. Fertil Steril. 2007; 87(4):858–61. S0015-0282(06)04386-X [pii]
17. Check JH, Nowroozi K, Chase JS, Nazari A, Shapse D, Vaze M. ovulation induction and pregnancies in 100 consecutive women with hypergonadotropic amenorrhea. Fertil Steril. 1990; 53(5):811–6.
18. Surrey ES, Cedars MI. The effect of gonadotropin suppression on the induction of ovulation in premature ovarian failure patients. Fertil Steril. 1989; 52(1):36–41.
19. Robles A, Checa MA, Prat M, Carreras R. Medical alternatives to oocyte donation in women with premature ovarian failure: A systematic review. Gynecol Endocrinol. 2013; 29(7):632–7. doi:10.3109/0951 3590.2013.797397
20. van Kasteren YM, Braat DD, Hemrika DJ, Lambalk CB, Rekers-Mombarg LT, von Blomberg BM et al. Corticosteroids do not influence ovarian responsiveness to gonadotropins in patients with premature ovarian failure: A randomized, placebo-controlled trial. Fertil Steril. 1999; 71(1):90–5. S0015028298004117 [pii]
21. Badawy A, Goda H, Ragab A. Induction of ovulation in idiopathic premature ovarian failure: A randomized double-blind trial. Reprod Biomed Online. 2007; 15(2):215–9.
22. Corenblum B, Rowe T, Taylor PJ. High-dose, short-term glucocorticoids for the treatment of infertility resulting from premature ovarian failure. Fertil Steril. 1993; 59(5):988–91.
23. Yeung TW, Li RH, Lee VC, Ho PC, Ng EH. A randomized double-blinded placebo-controlled trial on the effect of dehydroepiandrosterone for 16 weeks on ovarian response markers in women with primary ovarian insufficiency. J Clin Endocrinol Metab. 2013; 98(1):380–8. doi:10.1210/jc.2012-3071
24. Mamas L, Mamas E. Premature ovarian failure and dehydroepiandrosterone. Fertil Steril. 2009; 91(2):644–6. doi:10.1016/j.fertnstert.2007.11.055
25. Stoop D, Cobo A, Silber S. Fertility preservation for age-related fertility decline. Lancet. 2014; 384(9950):1311–9. doi:10.1016/S0140-6736(14)61261-7
26. Lutjen P, Trounson A, Leeton J, Findlay J, Wood C, Renou P. The establishment and maintenance of pregnancy using in vitro fertilization and embryo donation in a patient with primary ovarian failure. Nature. 1984; 307(5947):174–5.
27. Nelson SM, Lawlor DA. Predicting live birth, preterm delivery, and low birth weight in infants born from in vitro fertilisation: A prospective study of 144,018 treatment cycles. PLoS Med. 2011; 8(1):e1000386. doi:10.1371/journal.pmed.1000386
28. Tarlatzis BC, Pados G. Oocyte donation: Clinical and practical aspects. Mol Cell Endocrinol. 2000; 161(1–2):99–102. S0303-7207(99)00229-4 [pii]
29. Soderstrom-Anttila V, Tiitinen A, Foudila T, Hovatta O. Obstetric and perinatal outcome after oocyte donation: Comparison with in-vitro fertilization pregnancies. Hum Reprod. 1998; 13(2):483–90.
30. Antinori S, Gholami GH, Versaci C, Cerusico F, Dani L, Antinori M et al. Obstetric and prenatal outcome in menopausal women: A 12-year clinical study. Reprod Biomed Online. 2003; 6(2):257–61.
31. van Dorp W, Rietveld AM, Laven JS, van den Heuvel-Eibrink MM, Hukkelhoven CW, Schipper I. Pregnancy outcome of non-anonymous oocyte donation: A case-control study. Eur J Obstet Gynecol Reprod Biol. 2014; 182:107–12. doi:10.1016/j.ejogrb.2014.09.019
32. Stoop D, Baumgarten M, Haentjens P, Polyzos NP, De Vos M, Verheyen G et al. Obstetric outcome in donor oocyte pregnancies: A matched-pair analysis. Reprod Biol Endocrinol. 2012; 10:42-7827-10-42. doi:10.1186/1477-7827-10-42
33. Ameratunga D, Weston G, Osianlis T, Catt J, Vollenhoven B. In vitro fertilisation (IVF) with donor eggs in post-menopausal women: Are there differences in pregnancy outcomes in women with premature ovarian failure (POF) compared with women with physiological age-related menopause? J Assist Reprod Genet. 2009; 26(9–10):511–4. doi:10.1007/s10815-009-9351-5

34. van der Schouw YT, van der Graaf Y, Steyerberg EW, Eijkemans JC, Banga JD. Age at menopause as a risk factor for cardiovascular mortality. Lancet. 1996; 347(9003):714–8.

35. Hagman A, Loft A, Wennerholm UB, Pinborg A, Bergh C, Aittomaki K et al. Obstetric and neonatal outcome after oocyte donation in 106 women with Turner syndrome: A Nordic cohort study. Hum Reprod. 2013; 28(6):1598–609. doi:10.1093/humrep/det082

36. Awwad JT, Ghazeeri GS, Hannoun A, Isaacson K, Abou-Abdallah M, Farra CG. An investigational ovarian stimulation protocol increased significantly the psychological burden in women with premature ovarian failure. Acta Obstet Gynecol Scand. 2012; 91(11):1273–8. doi:10.1111/aogs.12004

22

How to Define Success in Ovulation Induction

Miriam Braakhekke, Madelon van Wely, and Ben W. Mol

Introduction

The aim of assisted reproductive techniques (ART) is to assist subfertile couples to achieve a pregnancy. There is a variety of ARTs, some of which aim to overcome a specific pathologic mechanism, and others simply aim to increase conception chances without targeting a cause, for example, in unexplained subfertility.

The definition of success of these treatments is obviously primarily driven by its aim, the birth of a healthy child. However, there are varieties on this theme. When a patient is known to have specific pathology, a treatment can be seen as successful when this pathologic mechanism is solved or bypassed. In women with anovulation, for example, ovulation induction aims to overcome a specific pathologic hurdle, anovulation. Induction of ovulation aims at monofollicular development, subsequent ovulation, singleton pregnancy, and ultimately the birth of a healthy newborn. In this chapter, we aim to give an overview on how to define success and complications of ovulation induction.

The WHO describes infertility as "a disease of the reproductive system defined by the failure to achieve a clinical pregnancy after 12 months or more of regular unprotected sexual intercourse." The 12 months mentioned in this description refer to 13 ovulations, and in women with ovulatory disorders, the number of ovulations is limited, thus reducing fertility chances.

Ovulatory disorders can have different underlying causes. The WHO differentiates three categories of women with anovulation (see also Chapter 2):

1. Hypogonadotropic hypogonadal anovulation
2. Normogonadotropic normoestrogenic anovulation
3. Hypergonadotropic hypoestrogenic anovulation

In WHO 2 anovulation, polycystic ovarian syndrome (PCOS) is the most common cause of anovulatory infertility as discussed in Chapter 5. We will continue this chapter presuming that we define the effectiveness of ovulation induction in women with PCOS.

Overview of Existing Evidence

Success in Ovulation Induction

Women who are trying to conceive and suffer from anovulation usually have a reasonable chance of conception when ovulations are induced, particularly when anovulation was the only cause of infertility. Approximately 75%–80% of women with anovulation based on PCOS who start ovulation induction with clomiphene citrate (CC) will ovulate, and about 50% will have conceived after six cycles (LOE 2a) (1). Thus, ovulation induction might be defined as successful when ovulation occurs, but this denies the underlying absence of having a child for almost half of the couples.

The PCOS consensus workgroup of ASRM and ESHRE advice is to continue ovulation induction with CC in PCOS for six cycles in which spontaneous conception can be achieved. The conventional treatment for women who ovulate on CC is therefore to continue for six treatment cycles; however, it is unclear how many additional cycles of treatment with CC are effective (LOE 2a) (2). Some couples might benefit from an earlier switch to a more aggressive treatment, for example, gonadotropins and/or intrauterine insemination (IUI), and others might benefit from continuation of the treatment for more than six cycles.

It is important to realize that medical treatments usually focus on the establishment of a single ovulation, which then provides the chance of subsequent conception. If conception does not occur, the treatment can only be successful through repetitive ovulation induction in subsequent cycles. Other treatments, however, such as lifestyle interventions or surgery, might establish ovulation in a more structural way. When lifestyle interventions result in a structural improvement of lifestyle, this might be effective over a multiple number of cycles (LOE 1a) (3) (see also Chapter 20). Similarly, surgical interventions, laparoscopic electrocoagulation of the ovaries (LEO) being the most established, also may result in multiple ovulations (LOE 1b) (4) (see also Chapter 18). Both treatments remain possibly effective even after the first pregnancy. In women with PCOS resistant to CC, for example, follow-up of a randomized comparison between LEO of the ovaries and treatment with recombinant FSH showed that women treated with surgery had larger families 10 years after randomization, probably due to the fact that women in the surgery group more often had a regular cycle after initial treatment, and women in the recombinant FSH group remained more often anovulatory without treatment (LOE 1b) (4).

Thus, the definition of success of ovulation induction has multiple dimensions, on the cycle level in terms of ovulation as well as pregnancy and live birth and on the reproductive life of the woman and her family. Apart from that, studies should report on harm for treatment and report on cost-effectiveness. Finally, it has become clear that women with anovulation, particularly PCOS, are at increased risk for other diseases, including cardiovascular risk and diabetes. The latter should also be considered.

Complications

In the choice of a treatment to reach the desired outcome, one should also consider potential disadvantages, including side effects. Different treatment options are, of course, related to different side effects at different time points of the treatment. In studies on ovulation induction, harms to all participants as well as side effects should be systematically collected and reported at all time points: during the intervention, during pregnancy, and in the long term.

During the Intervention

Clomiphene citrate tends to have a low chance of complications as only a few side effects are registered. Visual impairment is reported in 1.5% of the women that use clomiphene citrate. The incidence of multiple pregnancies is low, around 8% (LOE 2a) (5).

The use of gonadotrophins results in a higher risk of multiple pregnancies, up to 22%, and ovarian hyperstimulation syndrome might occur (LOE 1a) (6). Immediate complications of laparoscopic electrocoagulation of the ovaries are rare although hemorrhage and bowel perforation may occur.

During Pregnancy

Women with PCOS have a higher risk of gestational diabetes, pregnancy-induced hypertension, and preeclampsia (LOE 2a), which might also be caused by BMI, multiple pregnancy, and/or lower parity.

However, these complications are not associated with a particular treatment option for ovulation induction (7).

Long-Term Outcome

Later in life, women with PCOS have a significant risk of impaired glucose tolerance resulting in diabetes (LOE 2a). These risks are highest in women who have both oligo-ovulation and hyperandrogenism and are further increased by obesity. Many studies report that women with PCOS, whether lean or obese, have an increased cardiovascular risk profile with a higher blood pressure and abnormal lipid profile. These metabolic and cardiovascular diseases in women with PCOS are not affected by the way PCOS was treated earlier in life (7). Couples should thus be informed; however, it does not affect the choice for a particular treatment.

It has been suggested that laparoscopic electrocoagulation of the ovaries can lead to ovarian damage and adhesion formation and thus lead to premature ovarian failure and secondary infertility (8). Although, FSH as well as AMH levels after LEO seem to be, respectively, higher and lower, long-term follow up of women randomized between ovulation induction with gonadotropins and LEO showed no differences between the occurrence of premature ovarian failure. The need for assisted reproductive techniques in order to conceive a second time was lower in the LEO group (LOE 1b) (4).

Cost-Effectiveness

In economical evaluations, we consider not only effects of a treatment, but also the costs made during a specified time horizon, which in reproductive medicine, is usually 12 months. Reproductive medicine poses a challenge for health economists and policy makers. Fertility treatments are intrinsically different from other types of medical care because they are judged on their ability to create new life rather than to extend or improve the quality of existing life and therefore do not lend themselves to often used health economic methods. In cost-effectiveness analyses (CEA) in reproductive medicine, mostly pregnancy-related end points are used, such as clinical pregnancy, ongoing pregnancy, and delivery. These analyses take treatment costs and all costs up to the end point into consideration.

In ovulation induction, several studies have been performed to identify prognostic factors for treatment response. If prognostic factors are known, involving these factors in cost-effectiveness analyses can lead to patient-tailored treatment advice. In 2005, Eijkemans et al. tried to devise a patient-tailored, cost-effective treatment algorithm based on individual patient characteristics. They included age >30 years, amenorrhea, elevated androgen levels, and obesity as prognostic factors for treatment effect (9). The costs per pregnancy of three conventional strategies were compared, resulting in a cost-effective and patient-tailored advice.

To implement differences in safety profile of the treatments, cost-effectiveness analyses in reproductive medicine should include all pregnancy- and delivery-related costs. This is a minimum requirement of a useful CEA, but is it enough?

Knowledge of the effect of fertility treatments on development and health of children might also be crucial for a definite conclusion on the actual costs made by society (10). These child costs are more difficult to implement.

According to the NICE Fertility guidelines, economic evaluations should incorporate quality-adjusted life years or QALYs (11). A QALY measures improvements in health. Not cost-effectiveness, but cost utility is the primary method in doing so. Cost utility is used by policy makers as it allows for the economic comparison of interventions that result in different health outcomes as measured by QALYs. This is clearly not an easy task in fertility as QALYs are intended to capture improvements in health among living patients, and it is less straightforward to improve the health of someone who has not yet been conceived. More knowledge of the actual health and development of children conceived with fertility treatment will help us to create better estimates of the real live time costs.

Discussion

The issues stated above have impact on two levels of the assessment of effectiveness of ovulation induction. First, it influences the assessment of effectiveness within research. Second, it has impact on the counseling of couples in daily practice.

Assessment of Effectiveness of Ovulation Induction in Clinical Research

Clinical trials testing infertility treatments often do not report on the major outcomes of interest to patients, clinicians, and the public, live birth being the most important one.

In 2014, because of the inconsistencies in trial reporting, a group of investigators recommended that the preferred primary outcome of all infertility trials is live birth (defined as any delivery of a live infant ≥20 weeks gestation) or cumulative live birth (defined as the live birth per women over a defined time period or number of treatment cycles) (12).

For studies on ovulation induction, this does imply that studies on effectiveness of treatments should preferably compare the outcome over a larger number of cycles in a fixed period of time. Comparisons should explicitly report on a fixed period even if the number of cycles in that period differs between treatments. The intention-to-treat principle then accounts for the fact that on some treatments the actual ovulation induction should be compared.

Although live birth is considered to be the preferable outcome, we recommend that reports can limit themselves to the occurrence of ongoing pregnancy at 12 weeks gestation in a particular treatment period. This leads to the same conclusions, is less time- (and money-) consuming, and is less influenced by random error (LOE 2) (13,14).

Obviously, apart from pregnancy and live birth, studies should compare ovulation rates in studies. This is not only another measure for effectiveness; it also provides insight into the mechanism toward success of ovulation induction. In studies evaluating the effectiveness of ovulation induction, it is therefore also important to report on the mechanisms leading to pregnancy, that is, ovulation and conception. In the randomized trial of Legro et al., comparing letrozole and clomiphene citrate, the difference in live birth rate (27.5% vs. 19.1%) was partly explained by the difference in ovulation rate (61.7% vs. 48.3%) and partly by the difference in pregnancy rate conditional on conception (LOE 1b) (15). Thus, both measures should be reported on in infertility trials. Additionally, long-term follow-up of women should be recommended (LOE 4) (4).

Assessment of Effectiveness in the Counseling of Women

The above issues that count for evaluation of effectiveness in clinical studies obviously also count when treatments are discussed with couples. This preferably occurs in a model of shared decision making. Before the start of a treatment, the treatment strategy should be discussed with the patient. Important aspects include the aimed family size of the couple, willingness to undergo surgery, and preference for oral or subcutaneous medication. Side effects should be discussed at the same time (Figure 22.1).

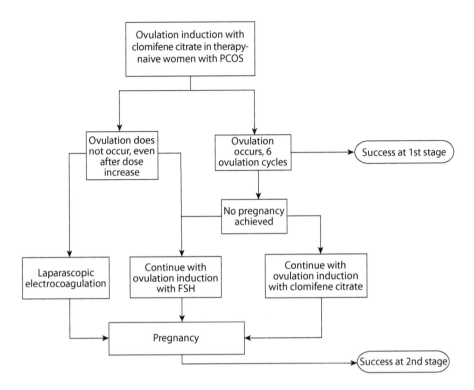

FIGURE 22.1 Success in ovulation induction. Long-term effects and complications should be part of counseling.

Conclusion

Subfertile couples suffering from anovulation should be well informed on treatment effect on the cycle level in terms of ovulation as well as pregnancy and live birth, on side effects, and on the reproductive life of the woman and her family, thus allowing shared decision making. Clinical research should follow this need. Studies assessing the effectiveness of ovulation induction in the short term should report on ovulation rates and on live birth over a multiple number of cycles. Preferably, studies should also assess short- as well as long-term (side) effects, including subsequent pregnancies and future cardiovascular health.

TABLE 22.1

Level of Evidence of Statements

Statement	Level of Evidence
Success of ovulation induction has multiple dimensions and depends on the stage and strategy of treatment.	2a
For cost-effectiveness analysis, fertility treatments are more difficult than for other types of medical care.	4
The definition of success of ovulation induction in clinical research can differ from the definition of success in daily practice.	4

TABLE 22.2

Grade of Strength for Recommendations

Recommendation	Grade Strength
Studies should report on multiple cycles on the outcomes of ovulation and ongoing pregnancy.	B
Couples should be well informed on treatment effect on the cycle level and on the reproductive life of the woman and her family.	C
Side effects at all time points should be considered.	C
Cost-effectiveness of ovulation induction might be patient-tailored, involving different prognostic factors.	D
After counseling of the couple, shared decision making is recommended.	D

REFERENCES

1. The Thessaloniki ESHRE/ASRM-Sponsored PCOS Consensus Workshop Group. Consensus on infertility treatment related to polycystic ovary syndrome. Hum Reprod [Internet]. 2008; 23(3):462–77. Available from: http://humrep.oxfordjournals.org/content/23/3/462.full.
2. Kousta E, White DM, Franks S. Modern use of clomiphene citrate in induction of ovulation. Hum Rep Update 1997; 3(4):359–65.
3. Moran LJ, Hutchison SK, Norman RJ, Teede HJ. Lifestyle changes in women with polycystic ovary syndrome. Cochrane Database Syst Rev. 2011; (7):CD007506.
4. Nahuis MJ, Kose N, Bayram N, van Dessel HJHM, Braat DDM, Hamilton CJCM et al. Long-term outcomes in women with polycystic ovary syndrome initially randomized to receive laparoscopic electrocautery of the ovaries or ovulation induction with gonadotrophins. Hum Reprod [Internet]. 2011 Jul [cited 2015 Jan 20]; 26(7):1899–904. Available from: http://www.ncbi.nlm.nih.gov/pubmed/21576081.
5. Brown J, Farquhar C, Beck J, Boothroyd C, Hughes E. Clomiphene and anti-oestrogens for ovulation induction in PCOS. Cochrane Database of Systematic Reviews. 2009; (4), Art. No.: CD002249.
6. Bayram N, van Wely M, Van der Veen F. Recombinant FSH versus urinary gonadotrophins or recombinant FSH for ovulation induction in subfertility associated with polycystic ovary syndrome. Cochrane Database of Systematic Reviews. 2001; (2), Art. No.: CD002121.
7. Marleen J. Nahuis, Eefje J. Oude Lohuis, Neriman Bayram, Peter G.A. Hompes, G. Jurjen E. Oosterhuis, Fulco van der Veen, Ben Willem J. Mol, Madelon van Wely. Pregnancy complications and metabolic disease in women with clomiphene citrate-resistant anovulation randomized to receive laparoscopic electrocautery of the ovaries or ovulation induction with gonadotropins: A 10-year follow-up. Fertility and Sterility. 2014; 101(1):270–274.
8. Kandil M, Selim M. Hormonal and sonographic assessment of ovarian reserve before and after laparoscopic ovarian drilling in polycystic ovary syndrome. BJOG An Int J Obstet Gynaecol. 2005; 112(10):1427–30.
9. Eijkemans MJC, Polinder S, Mulders AMGJ, Laven JSE, Habbema JDF, Fauser BCJM. Individualized cost-effective conventional ovulation induction treatment in normogonadotrophic anovulatory infertility (WHO group 2). Hum Reprod. 2005; 20(10):2830–7.
10. Chambers GM, Adamson GD, Eijkemans MJC. Acceptable cost for the patient and society. Fertil Steril [Internet]. Elsevier Inc.; 2013 Aug [cited 2015 Jan 20]; 100(2):319–27. Available from: http://www.ncbi.nlm.nih.gov/pubmed/23905708.
11. Fertility problems: Assessment and treatment. NICE guidelines [CG156]. February 2013.
12. Harbin Consensus Conference Workshop Group, Improving the Reporting of Clinical Trials of Infertility Treatments (IMPRINT): Modifying the CONSORT statement. Fertility and Sterility. 2014; 102(4):952–959.
13. Braakhekke M, Esme I. Kamphuis, Eline A. Dancet, Femke Mol, Fulco van der Veen, Ben W. Mol, Ongoing pregnancy qualifies best as the primary outcome measure of choice in trials in reproductive medicine: An opinion paper. Fertility and Sterility. 2014; 101(5):1203–4.
14. Clarke JF, van Rumste MME, Farquhar CM, Johnson NP, Mol BWJ, Herbison P. Measuring outcomes in fertility trials: Can we rely on clinical pregnancy rates? Fertil Steril [Internet]. Elsevier Ltd; 2010 Oct [cited 2013 Oct 23]; 94(5):1647–51. Available from: http://www.ncbi.nlm.nih.gov/pubmed/20056216.
15. Legro RS, Brzyski RG, Diamond MP, Coutifaris C, Schlaff WD, Casson P et al. Letrozole versus clomiphene for infertility in the polycystic ovary syndrome. N Engl J Med. 2014; 371:119–29.

23

Complications of Ovarian Stimulation: Multifollicular Development

Evert J. P. van Santbrink

Introduction

Ovarian stimulation in patients with chronic anovulation, traditionally classified as WHO classes 1 and 2 (see Chapters 14 through 16), is aiming at restoration of physiology: monthly follicular maturation and ovulation of a single dominant oocyte.

Conventional treatment is considered to be administration of gonadotropin-releasing hormone agonist (GnRH-agonist) or gonadotropins in WHO 1 anovulation and anti-estrogen (clomiphene citrate) followed, in case of treatment failure, by exogenous follicle-stimulating hormone (FSH) in WHO 2 patients. More recently, aromatase inhibitors as a new ovulation induction compound have been introduced for treatment of WHO 2 anovulation.

Regardless of the means used, it is often hard to control ovarian stimulation, resulting in multiple follicle development and ovulation. This may enable chances for complications, such as multiple pregnancy and ovarian hyperstimulation syndrome.

Although multiple follicle development will improve chances of a pregnancy, ovarian stimulation should be discontinued or conception prevented when chances of complications, that is, multiple pregnancy and ovarian hyperstimulation syndrome (OHSS), are too high.

Overview of Existing Evidence

Prevention of Multifollicular Growth

In general, it can be stated that the risk of complications in ovulation induction can be reduced by an individualized treatment schedule, frequent treatment monitoring, and strict cancellation criteria (LOE 4).

GnRH

In WHO 1 anovulation with intact pituitary function, administration of pulsatile GnRH-agonist can restore ovulation (Chapter 14). Although the hormonal feedback loop between pituitary and ovaries remains functional, chances of multifollicular growth and concomitant complications are low (LOE 3). In a relatively large study population, multiple pregnancy rate was 3.2%, and no OHSS was reported (1).

Anti-Estrogens/Aromatase Inhibitors

Possibilities for prevention of multifollicular development during ovulation induction in WHO 2 anovulation using anti-estrogens or aromatase inhibitors are limited: These drugs are administered mostly from day 3 to day 7 after the start of a spontaneous or progestogen-induced withdrawal bleeding. The effect of this treatment can only be determined afterwards, so there is no correction possible during the treatment cycle. Therefore, treatment is started with a low daily dose, which may be increased in a following treatment cycle in case of absence of adequate ovarian response. Although reported chances on complications after ovulation induction with anti-estrogens or aromatase inhibitors are low (LOE 3), one could accept this as a calculated risk without monitoring or decide to prevent conception in case of multi-follicular development during ultrasound or serum estrogen monitoring (Chapters 24 and 25).

Gonadotropins (FSH)

Gonadotropins may be used for ovulation induction in WHO 1 and WHO 2 anovulation. The extended half-life of FSH makes it hard to predict how many follicles are going to reach the dominant status, and sometimes, daily ovarian ultrasound monitoring is required to adjust the treatment dosage before multifollicular development is a fact. This may result in daily hospital visits and increased patient inconvenience.

To prevent multifollicular growth, it is essential to surpass the FSH threshold for such a restricted period that only one follicle is allowed into ongoing development and dominance (2). This may be accomplished by a low-dose regimen in which the daily FSH dose is changed in small increments (25–37 IU) at 5- to 7-day intervals (Chapter 19).

Using frequent monitoring and strict cancellation criteria during a low-dose step-up gonadotropin stimulation protocol may result in 70%–80% monofollicular development (1 follicle ≥ 16 mm) and 15%–18% cancellation rate of all started treatment cycles (White 1996; 3) (LOE 3).

An alternative way to monitor follicle development during ovulation induction may be measurement of circulating estradiol concentrations. Although the ASRM Practice Committee recommends caution when serum estradiol is rising rapidly or exceeds 2500 pg/ml in a recent study, a much lower threshold of 400 pg/ml is recommended (4). In regard to the aim of ovulation induction, that is, single follicle development, the 400 pg/ml threshold may be a more realistic cancellation criterion (Chapter 25).

Before starting FSH ovulation induction, chances for multifollicular development could be predicted by initial patient characteristics, such as hyperandrogenism (increased serum AD and T), elevated luteinizing hormone (LH), and increased antral follicle count (5). So it may be more difficult to accomplish monofollicular development in patients with a more explicit PCOS phenotype (LOE 3). This may be taken into account while setting up an individualized treatment schedule to optimize results and lower complications (6).

A completely different possibility to normalize ovarian response to hormonal stimulation and therefore decrease chances of multifollicular development is alteration of the endocrine milieu (LOE 2). This may be performed using lifestyle interventions (weight reduction), insulin sensitizers, or laparoscopic electrocautery of the ovaries (LEO). This is discussed in Chapters 17, 18, and 20.

Management of Multifollicular Growth

When multifollicular development is determined during monitoring of ovulation induction, chances for multiple pregnancy and ovarian hyperstimulation syndrome (OHSS) are increased. From studies in patients treated for ovulation induction (clomiphene as well as gonadotropins) and controlled ovarian hyperstimulation in combination with IUI, it is reported that there is a significant increase in multiple pregnancy rate when, on the day of hCG administration, there were at least two follicles of ≥13 mm diameter or a serum estradiol > 400 pg/L (4,7) (LOE 3).

In the management of multifollicular development, there should be a balance between the chance to reach the treatment goal (i.e., ongoing pregnancy) and the complication risk. This balance contains, besides a medical risk, an individual patient choice; therefore, this should be discussed extensively with every patient before treatment is started.

Conclusion

It may be concluded that the risk of multiple follicle development in ovulation induction using a GnRH agonist, anti-estrogen, or aromatase inhibitor is low. However, in gonadotropin ovulation induction, ovarian response is hard to predict, and multiple development is far more probable to occur. Frequent monitoring, individualized treatment programs, and strict cancellation criteria are mandatory to prevent this.

TABLE 23.1

Level of Evidence of Statements

Statement	Level of Evidence
The purpose of ovulation induction is monofollicular growth and ovulation.	3
Multiple follicular development is associated with increased chances of (multiple) pregnancy.	1a
During ovulation induction, the chance of multiple follicle development is reduced by frequent monitoring and strict cancellation criteria.	3/4
Ultrasound as well as serum estradiol measurement can be utilized for monitoring follicle development during ovulation induction.	3
Low-dose gonadotropin protocols in ovulation induction decrease risk of multiple follicle development.	3
It is more difficult to accomplish monofollicular development in a patient with a more explicit PCOS phenotype.	3
Changes in endocrine milieu can decrease chances of multiple follicle development in ovulation induction.	1b
Using frequent monitoring and strict cancellation criteria during a low-dose step-up gonadotropin stimulation protocol results in 70%–80% monofollicular development.	3

TABLE 23.2

Grade of Strength for Recommendations

Recommendation	Grade Strength
The aim of ovulation induction is monofollicular development.	C
Frequent monitoring and strict cancellation criteria are mandatory to prevent multiple follicle development.	B
A low-dose gonadotropin stimulation protocol should be used instead of a high-dose protocol, to reduce the complication risk.	B
The patient should be counseled about the multiple pregnancy risk before treatment starts.	D

REFERENCES

1. Filicori M, Flamigni C, Dellai P et al. Treatment of anovulation with pulsatile GnRH: Prognostic factors and clinical results in 600 cycles. J Clin Endocrinol Metab 1994; 79:1215–20.
2. White DM, Polson DW, Kiddy D et al. Induction of ovulation with low-dose gonadotropins in polycystic ovary syndrome: An analysis of 109 pregnancies in 225 women. J Clin Endocrinol Metab 1996; 81:3821–4.
3. van Santbrink EJ, Fauser BC. Is there a future tor ovulation induction in the current era of assisted reproduction? Hum Reprod 2003; 18(12):2499–502.
4. Goldman RH, Batsis M, Petrozza JC, Souter I. Patient-specific predictions of outcome after gonadotropin ovulation induction/intrauterine insemination. Fertil Steril 2014; 101(6):1649–55.
5. Mulders, AG et al. Prediction of chances for success or complications in gonadotrophin ovulation induction in normogonadotrophic anovulatory infertility. Reprod Biomed Onl 2003; 7:170–8.
6. van Santbrink EJ, Eijkemans MJ, Laven SJ et al. Patient-tailored conventional ovulation induction algorithms in anovulatory infertility. Trends Endocrinol Metab 2005; 16:381–9.
7. van Rumste MM, Custers IM, van der Veen F, van Wely M, Evers JL, Mol BW. The influence of the number of follicles on pregnancy rates in intrauterine insemination with ovarian stimulation: A meta-analysis. Hum Reprod Update 2008; 14(6):563–70.

24

Complications of Ovulation Induction: Ovarian Hyperstimulation Syndrome

Botros Rizk and Miriam Baumgarten

Introduction

Ovarian hyperstimulation syndrome (OHSS) is a condition inherently related to controlled ovarian stimulation.

It can, however, occur in a spontaneous ovulatory cycle. The underlying mechanism of this rarity is believed to be related to a mutation in the FSH receptor (1). Typically, OHSS occurs as an iatrogenic complication in women undergoing IVF/ICSI due to the supra-physiological doses of gonadotrophins, which are used to induce multifollicular growth. OHSS is a clinical diagnosis based on symptoms. The majority of these symptoms are a result of increased vascular permeability of the gonadotropin-primed ovaries. The syndrome can be best characterized by bilaterally enlarged ovaries due to multiple follicular and thecal lutein ovarian cysts. In addition to the physical enlargement of ovaries, an acute shift of intravascular fluid distribution occurs, causing clinical ascites, leading to serious complications and, ultimately, death (2–5).

The accurate incidence of OHSS is difficult to state because of the different classifications used in the literature. The incidence varies between patient groups and treatments used. In IVF, up to 33% of cycles develop mild OHSS. Although they are considered clinically less significant, they still have the potential to develop into the severe form, which is estimated to occur in 3.1%–8.0% of cycles (6).

The development of OHSS with ovulation induction using gonadotropins or clomiphene citrate is even less well studied. Anecdotal cases can be found in the literature, but the true incidence is unknown (7,8).

Classification of OHSS

OHSS may be mild, moderate, or severe; early or late in onset; spontaneous or iatrogenic in etiology.

Early OHSS presents 3 to 7 days after the trigger to induce ovulation whereas late OHSS presents 12 to 17 days after ovulation. Early OHSS relates to "excessive" pre-ovulatory response to stimulation whereas late OHSS depends on the occurrence of pregnancy, is more likely to be severe, and is only poorly related to pre-ovulatory events.

There has been no unanimity in classifying OHSS, and divergent classifications have made comparisons between studies difficult. In 1999, Rizk and Aboulghar introduced a classification dividing the syndrome into moderate (group B) and severe (group C) with the purpose of categorizing patients into more defined clinical groups, which correlate with the prognosis of the syndrome. The new classification can be correlated with the treatment protocol and prognosis (9). The mild degree (group A) of OHSS, used by most previous authors was omitted from the new classification as this degree occurs in the majority of cases of ovarian stimulation and does not require special treatment. The great majority of cases of

TABLE 24.3

Classification of Severity of OHSS (RCOG Guideline No. 5)

Grade	Symptoms
Mild OHSS	Abdominal bloating
	Mild abdominal pain
	Ovarian size usually less than 8 cm
Moderate OHSS	Moderate abdominal pain
	Nausea with or without vomiting
	Ultrasound evidence of ascites
	Ovarian size usually 8–12 cm
Severe OHSS	Clinical ascites (occasionally hydrothorax)
	Oliguria
	Hemoconcentration with a hematocrit >45%
	Hypoproteinemia
	Ovarian size usually more than 12 cm
Critical OHSS	Tense ascites or large hydrothorax
	Hematocrit >55%
	White cell count >25,000/ml
	Oliguria or anuria
	Thromboembolism
	Acute respiratory syndrome

OHSS with ovulation induction present with symptoms belonging to category of mild OHSS. During clomiphene citrate ovulation induction cycles, the incidence of mild OHSS might be seen in up to 13% of cycles (10). ESHRE and the ASRM also support this classification categorizing OHSS into mild, moderate, and severe forms.

The Royal College of Obstetricians and Gynaecologists (RCOG), through its Guideline and Audit Committee and Professional Standards Committee, produces Clinical Governance guidance documents for gynecologists practicing in the United Kingdom. This provides us with a classification and advice on appropriate treatment. With the reflection on mild and moderate OHSS classification, modified as suggested by Mathur in 2005 (11). Table 24.3 is the used classification of severity of OHSS in the United Kingdom with the footnote that ovarian size may not correlate with severity of OHSS in cases of assisted reproduction because of the effect of follicular aspiration.

Prediction of OHSS

Prediction of OHSS is the cornerstone of prevention. Prediction is based on identifying the characteristics of the patients who would be high responders for primary prevention as well as identifying the patient at risk during stimulation.

Patient characteristics of women at risk for OHSS mentioned in literature are previous OHSS, youth, low BMI, PCO(S), high AMH, and single nucleotide polymorphism for FSH-R, LH-R, E2-R, and AMH-R (12).

For secondary prevention ultrasonography and estradiol assessment during stimulation can be used. A rapid rise of estradiol or a high serum level (4000 pg/ml) are associated with over-response (13,14).

Ultrasound is widely used for monitoring follicular development in assisted conception (see also Chapter 21). The number, size, and pattern of distribution of the follicles are important in the prediction of OHSS (9). The diagnosis of polycystic ovaries at ultrasound examination (the necklace sign) improved the prediction of OHSS to 79% (15). Also, it was stated that a decrease in the fraction of mature follicles and an increase in the fraction of very small follicles correlated with an augmented risk for the development of severe OHSS (16). Additionally, there was a significant correlation between the baseline ovarian volume and the subsequent occurrence of OHSS 13.2+/15 ml versus 8.9+/-3.7 ml ($P = 0.035$), suggesting that volumetry of the ovaries could help to detect patients at risk of developing OHSS in case of stimulation for IVF (17). Keeping in mind that all these studies were about ovarian stimulation for

IVF, the actual predictive value of these tests are difficult to extrapolate to ovulation induction. One can, however, hypothesize that predicting the patients at risk for OHSS is comparable to the ones doing so during ovulation induction.

Checa et al. concluded, in a small prospective study, that an antral follicle count of 16 is predictive (sensitivity of 100%, specificity of 93%) for exacerbated response leading to cycle cancellation not commenting on OHSS (18).

In the majority of studies regarding ovulation induction, the under- or over-response is examined and not OHSS. The link between clomiphene citrate over-response or clomiphene citrate resistance and the response to gonadotropins needs to be explored. Our own unpublished experience with PCOS patients showed clomiphene citrate resistance is associated with over-response using standard ovarian stimulation for IVF.

Patients who hyper-responded on clomiphene citrate are likely to over-respond to ovarian stimulation and would therefore be classified as being at risk for OHSS. The response to clomiphene citrate depends on metabolism; therefore, the response to exogenous FSH cannot directly be correlated.

Prevention of Ovarian Hyperstimulation Syndrome

Laparoscopic Ovarian Drilling in PCOS Patients (See Also Chapter 16)

As previously mentioned, women suffering from PCOS are a challenging group. The threshold beyond which women over-respond to stimulation is difficult to determine. In reviews looking at ovarian drilling for ovulation induction and the efficacy, there is no difference in live birth rate (19). There is, however, no data on OHSS.

Laparoscopic ovarian drilling has been used successfully for prevention of OHSS in patients with polycystic ovaries undergoing IVF (20).

As ovarian drilling can make clomiphene citrate–resistant ovaries more susceptible for stimulation; needing less aggressive stimulation will reduce the risk of developing OHSS in theory (LOE 4).

Metformin

Short-term co-treatment with metformin for patients with PCOS undergoing IVF/ICSI cycles does not improve the response to stimulation but significantly improves the pregnancy outcome and reduces the risk of OHSS (21). No data is available for ovulation induction with metformin and a potential reduction of OHSS.

Cancel Cycle/Withhold hCG

As identifying the few patients who will develop OHSS with ovulation induction is so difficult, we can only focus on secondary prevention. This is when we diagnose over-response.

In order to prevent the angiogenesis of the follicles leading to the syndrome, ovulation should be avoided. Administration of hCG as an ovulation trigger is likely to have a negative effect and should be avoided in hyper-response. The couples should be advised to refrain from intercourse as the development of a pregnancy, especially a multiple pregnancy, will further stimulate the ovaries. Two to ten percent of IUI cycles get cancelled due to mild OHSS (10). One Indian series was found after extensive search of the literature. The authors report 1000 cycles of ovulation induction with the combination of clomiphene citrate and gonadotropins. They have 320 cycles with mild OHSS (abdominal pain and enlarged ovaries). Seventeen cycles developed moderate OHSS, 15 after trigger. Eleven cycles were cancelled, and four converted to IVF (22) (LOE-4).

In daily practice, late-onset OHSS with ovulation induction is probably seen most in PCOS patients.

Hypothesizing that the large amount of follicles in the presence of a pregnancy have increased permeability. The majority of the patients we see have enlarged ovaries and some free fluid and maybe some mild abdominal discomfort. As these are common symptoms in early pregnancy, as is ultrasound-found free fluid, no records of incidence are freely available.

Intravenous Albumin and HES

Experience in subjects with different forms of third space fluid accumulation have shown that albumin is efficacious in preventing and correcting hemodynamic instability. It acts to sequester vasoactive substances released from the corpora lutea, and the oncotic properties of albumin serve to maintain intravascular volume and prevent the ensuing effects of hypovolemia, ascites, and hemoconcentration.

Hydroxyethyl starch (HES) markedly decreased the incidence of severe OHSS. There was limited evidence of borderline benefit for intravenous albumin administration (23).

In IVF, this is done at the time of the egg collection, which routinely is 36 hours after the trigger injection. In case of over-response with ovulation induction, theoretically an infusion can be given after the assumed ovulation. There is, however, no evidence this would prevent women from developing symptoms. With ovulation induction combined with IUI, this would be the time of administration. A slow infusion of 1 L 6% HES is the most quoted protocol (LOE 3).

Rescue IVF/GnRH Agonist Trigger

In case of the development of multiple follicles, another option than completely cancelling the cycle is converting the cycle to rescue IVF.

A few studies have been done looking at the outcome of these cycles. Pregnancy rates are acceptable, and compared to conventional IVF, it is cost-effective. No cases of OHSS were described (24–27).

No randomized studies are available, nor is there an optimal protocol established. When the ovulation induction is started with clomiphene citrate, FSH can be added to add follicular development. In case the ovulation induction is started with gonadotropins, increasing the dose can be considered. A GnRH antagonist should be added to prevent premature ovulation. To avoid OHSS, the best trigger is a GnRH agonist (28). This can also be considered when not performing an oocyte retrieval. Pregnancy rates after a GnRH agonist trigger are lower due to a luteal phase deficiency (29). Freezing all embryos and replacing them in a subsequent cycle would be a valid strategy.

Cantineau et al. published a Cochrane review in 2014 in which OHSS was encompassed as an adverse outcome of IUI treatment (30). The OHSS rate was stated in five studies (31–35).

OHSS rates were compared for hCG versus GnRH-a, and there was no evidence of a difference between groups (OR 2.27, 95% CI 0.65 to 7.91; three trials, 456 women, low-quality evidence) (34,35). Shalev et al. reported four treatment cycles with grade three to grade four OHSS in the GnRH-a group and eight treatment cycles with OHSS in the hCG group; the other two studies in this meta-analysis reported none in either group (LOE 2).

The two studies comparing u-hCG with r-hCG for timing IUI reported no cases of (severe) OHSS in a total of 468 cycles (moderate-quality evidence) (31,33).

Dopamine Agonists in the Prevention/Treatment of OHSS

The use of a dopamine agonist has been studied with women suffering from over-response in IVF.

There are no data available about the use of dopamine agonists with OHSS due to ovulation induction. But taking into account the mechanism of action is to prevent extravasation of fluid, this treatment option can be offered to ovulation induction patients suffering from OHSS.

Vascular endothelial growth factor (VEGF) is a medicate of hCG-dependent ovarian angiogenesis. It induces endometrial cell proliferation and increases capillary permeability. VEGF is expressed in human ovaries (36), and its mRNA expression increases in granulosa cells after hCG administration (37).

Dopamine agonists, such as cabergoline, quinagolide, and bromocriptine, in vitro activate the dopamine receptor-2, promoting internalization of VEGFR-2 (becoming unreachable for VEGF) (38). In animal studies, phosphorylation of VEGFR induced by 42%, and the VGF production in cultured granulosa cells was exposed to hCG (39,40).

There are no studies about dopamine agonists in ovulation induction, but it has been used. Dopamine agonists might be beneficial to prevent symptoms of early nonsevere OHSS in IVF treatment (41).

The most quoted treatment protocol is 0.5 mg cabergoline for 8 days starting on the day of ovulation (LOE 3).

Treatment of Ovarian Hyperstimulation Syndrome

The clinical course of OHSS is determined by its severity, whether complications already occurred, and the presence or absence of pregnancy. The clinical management may involve dealing with electrolytic imbalance, neurohormonal and hemodynamic changes, pulmonary manifestation, liver dysfunction, hypoglobulinemia, febrile morbidity, thromboembolic phenomena, neurological manifestations, and adnexal torsion. Specific invasive approaches, such as abdominal or pleural paracentesis, should be carefully performed when necessary.

Outpatient Management for Moderate OHSS

Moderate OHSS can be followed up on an outpatient basis. This depends if a dedicated unit is able to provide this service (24/7) and if the patient is compliant.

A proposed treatment protocol would involve regular phone calls with the patient and a visit to the unit twice a week.

During the clinical assessment, the reported symptoms are most important, but additional tests can be performed. Following the ovarian size and the amount of free fluid can indicate if the syndrome is resolving.

It is important to provide support to the patient. Explain the self-limiting nature of the syndrome. Of unpublished own data, a patient questionnaire given to patients with OHSS after IVF found the abdominal swelling one of the most distressing symptoms.

Ovarian size can be measured in the three planes, or if available, an accurate volume can be obtained using 3-D ultrasound. Depending on the size of the ovaries, the use of vaginal or abdominal approach can be decided.

A full blood count with clotting will give biological information of the risk of thrombosis.

Patients should be instructed to contact the unit at any point when they have not passed urine for 12 hours, if they experience problems breathing, or with any other concern.

Circulatory Volume Correction

The main line of treatment is correction of the circulatory volume and the electrolyte imbalance. Every effort should be directed toward restoring a normal intravascular volume and preserving adequate renal function. Volume replacement should begin with intravenous crystalloid fluids at 125–150 ml/h. Normal saline and lactated Ringer have been successfully used. Plasma colloid expanders may be used if necessary. One concern with using plasma expanders is that the beneficial effect is transitory before their redistribution into the extravascular space, further exacerbating ascite formation.

Anticoagulant Treatment/Prophylaxis

Anticoagulant therapy is indicated if there is clinical evidence of thrombosis or if hematocrit is more than 45% (LOE 3). Venous thrombosis is the most common serious complication of OHSS. Preventive treatment with low molecular heparin should be used whenever there is a thromboembolic risk. In cases of severe OHSS, the following situations are recognized as indicating an increased risk of thromboembolism: immobilization, compression of pelvic vessels by large ovaries or ascites, pregnancy coagulation abnormalities, and hyperestrogenemia. Prevention using mobilization and antithrombotic stockings are insufficient as thrombosis may occur at all localizations and may be systemic in nature. Prophylaxis with heparin remains debatable for the reasons that there are no randomized studies proving its efficacy in preventing thromboembolic complications during severe OHSS. Despite these reservations, we recommend giving fractionated or low molecular weight heparin for patients with severe OHSS.

Conclusion

To prevent OHSS during ovulation induction, preventing ovulation might be the key!

TABLE 24.1

Level of Evidence of Statements

Statement	Level of Evidence
OHSS with ovulation induction is a rare complication.	2b
Women with PCOS or previous OHSS can be identified as women at risk of developing OHSS with ovulation induction.	4
Prevent OHSS by using a step-up protocol for ovulation induction with gonodotrophin.	2b
u-hCG versus rec-hCG trigger does not increase OHSS for ovulation induction combined with IUI.	2a
Trigger with GnRH analog reduced OHSS compared to hCG.	2a
HES 6% infusion during the time of IUI when ultrasound free fluid is present can prevent OHSS symptoms.	4
Rescue IVF is a valid option in case of over-response to prevent the development of OHSS.	3
Dopamine agonists might be useful for reducing OHSS symptoms, but the evidence is limited.	2b

TABLE 24.2

Grade of Strength for Recommendations

Recommendation	Grade Strength
Consider ovarian drilling for POCS patients.	D
Prophylactic LMWH in case of OHSS.	GPP
Secondary prevention involves cycle cancellation with or without GnRH antagonist treatment and cabergoline.	D
In over-response, use an GnHR agonist trigger and convert to IVF with freeze-all embryos.	D

REFERENCES

1. Dieterich M, Bolz M, Reimer T, Costagliola S, Gerber B. Two different entities of spontaneous ovarian hyperstimulation in a woman with FSH receptor mutation. Reprod Biomed Online. 20(6):751–8.
2. Beerendonk CC, van Dop PA, Braat DD, Merkus JM. Ovarian hyperstimulation syndrome: Facts and fallacies. Obstet Gynecol Surv. 53(7):439–49.
3. Mozes M, Bogokowsky H, Antebi E, Lunenfeld B, Rabau E, Serr DM et al. Thromboembolic phenomena after ovarian stimulation with human gonadotrophins. Lancet. 1965; 2(7424):1213–5.
4. Semba S, Moriya T, Youssef EM, Sasano H. An autopsy case of ovarian hyperstimulation syndrome with massive pulmonary edema and pleural effusion. Pathol Int. 50(7):549–52.
5. Cluroe AD, Synek BJ. A fatal case of ovarian hyperstimulation syndrome with cerebral infarction. Pathology. 1995; 27(4):344–6.
6. Delvigne A, Rozenberg S. Epidemiology and prevention of ovarian hyperstimulation syndrome (OHSS): A review. Hum Reprod Update. 8(6):559–77.
7. Thakur R, El-Menabawey M. Combined intra-uterine and extra-uterine pregnancy associated with mild hyperstimulation syndrome after clomiphene ovulation induction. Hum Reprod. 1996; 11(7):1583–4.
8. Abbas SM, Rouzi AA. Pregnancy with 15 live fetuses and severe ovarian hyperstimulation syndrome after ovulation induction and intrauterine insemination. Clin Exp Obstet Gynecol. 2013; 40(2):297–9.
9. Rizk B, Aboulghar M. Modern management of ovarian hyperstimulation syndrome. Hum Reprod. 6(8):1082–7.
10. Cantineau AE, Cohlen BJ, Heineman MJ. Ovarian stimulation protocols (anti-oestrogens, gonadotrophins with and without GnRH agonists/antagonists) for intrauterine insemination (IUI) in women with subfertility. Cochrane Database Syst Rev. 2007; (2):Cd005356.
11. Mathur R, Evboumwan I, Jenkins J. Prevention and management of ovarian hyperstimulation syndrome. Curr Obstet Gynaecol. 2005; 15:132–8.
12. Humaidan P, Quartarolo J, Papanikolaou EG. Preventing ovarian hyperstimulation syndrome: Guidance for the clinician. Fertil Steril. 94(2):389–400.

13. Papanikolaou EG, Pozzobon C, Kolibianakis EM, Camus M, Tournaye H, Fatemi HM et al. Incidence and prediction of ovarian hyperstimulation syndrome in women undergoing gonadotropin-releasing hormone antagonist in vitro fertilization cycles. Fertil Steril. 2006; 85(1):112–20.

14. Aboulghar MA, Mansour RT. Ovarian hyperstimulation syndrome: Classifications and critical analysis of preventive measures. Hum Reprod Update. 9(3):275–89.

15. Delvigne A, Demoulin A, Smitz J, Donnez J, Koninckx P, Dhont M et al. The ovarian hyperstimulation syndrome in in-vitro fertilization: A Belgian multicentric study. I. clinical and biological features. Hum Reprod. 8(9):1353–60.

16. Tal J, Paz B, Samberg I, Lazarov N, Sharf M. Ultrasonographic and clinical correlates of menotropin versus sequential clomiphene citrate: Menotropin therapy for induction of ovulation. Fertil Steril. 1985; 44(3):342–9.

17. Danninger B, Brunner M, Obruca A, Feichtinger W. Prediction of ovarian hyperstimulation syndrome by ultrasound volumetric assessment [corrected] of baseline ovarian volume prior to stimulation. Hum Reprod. 1996; 11(8):1597–9.

18. Checa MA, Prat M, Carreras R. Antral follicle count as a predictor of hyperresponse in controlled ovarian hyperstimulation/intrauterine insemination in unexplained sterility. Fertil Steril. 2010; 94(3):1105–7.

22. Jain S, Agarwal J, Bhaskar J, Saxena A, Parihar AS. Medical management of ovarian hyperstimulation syndrome (OHSS) in 1500 IUI cycles. 2014.

23. Youssef MA, Al-Inany HG, Evers JL, Aboulghar M. Intra-venous fluids for the prevention of severe ovarian hyperstimulation syndrome. Cochrane Database Syst Rev. 2011; (2):Cd001302.

24. Balayla J, Granger L, St-Michel P, Villeneuve M, Fontaine JY, Desrosiers P et al. Rescue in vitro fertilization using a GnRH antagonist in hyper-responders from gonadotropin intrauterine insemination (IUI) cycles. J Assist Reprod Genet. 2013; 30(6):773–8.

25. Olufowobi O, Sharif K, Papaioannou S, Mohamed H, Neelakantan D, Afnan M. Role of rescue IVF-ET treatment in the management of high response in stimulated IUI cycles. J Obstet Gynaecol. 2005; 25(2):166–8.

26. Saleh, SE, Taha Ismail M, Elshmaa NS. The efficacy of converting high response—Ovulation induction cycles to in vitro fertilization in patients with PCOS. Middle East Fertil Soc J. 2014; 19(1):51–6.

27. Chimote AN, Chimote BN, Chimote NN, Nath NM, Chimote NM. editors. P-426—High response to Clomiphen citrate in intrauterine insemination cycles when converted into "rescue" IVF results in higher implantation rates compared to minimal stimulation IVF cycles. ESHRE; 2015.

28. Humaidan P, Kol S, Papanikolaou EG. GnRH agonist for triggering of final oocyte maturation: Time for a change of practice? Human Reprod Update. 2011; 17(4):510–24.

29. Engmann L, Benadiva C, Humaidan P. GnRH agonist trigger for the induction of oocyte maturation in GnRH antagonist IVF cycles: A SWOT analysis. Reprod Biomed Online. 2016.

30. Cantineau AE, Janssen MJ, Cohlen BJ, Allersma T. Synchronised approach for intrauterine insemination in subfertile couples. Cochrane Database Syst Rev. 2014; 12:Cd006942.

31. Lorusso F, Palmisano M, Serrati G, Bassi E, Lamanna G, Vacca M et al. Intrauterine insemination with recombinant or urinary human chorionic gonadotropin: A prospective randomized trial. Gynecol Endocrinol. 2008; 24(11):644–8.

32. Martinez AR, Bernardus RE, Voorhorst FJ, Vermeiden JP, Schoemaker J. Pregnancy rates after timed intercourse or intrauterine insemination after human menopausal gonadotropin stimulation of normal ovulatory cycles: A controlled study. Fertil Steril. 1991; 55(2):258–65.

33. Sakhel K, Khedr M, Schwark S, Ashraf M, Fakih MH, Abuzeid M. Comparison of urinary and recombinant human chorionic gonadotropin during ovulation induction in intrauterine insemination cycles: A prospective randomized clinical trial. Fertil Steril. 2007; 87(6):1357–62.

34. Schmidt-Sarosi C, Kaplan DR, Sarosi P, Essig MN, Licciardi FL, Keltz M et al. Ovulation triggering in clomiphene citrate-stimulated cycles: Human chorionic gonadotropin versus a gonadotropin releasing hormone agonist. J Assist Reprod Genet. 1995; 12(3):167–74.

35. Shalev E, Geslevich Y, Matilsky M, Ben-Ami M. Induction of pre-ovulatory gonadotrophin surge with gonadotrophin-releasing hormone agonist compared to pre-ovulatory injection of human chorionic gonadotrophins for ovulation induction in intrauterine insemination treatment cycles. Hum Reprod. 1995; 10(9):2244–7.

36. Yan Z, Weich HA, Bernart W, Breckwoldt M, Neulen J. Vascular endothelial growth factor (VEGF) messenger ribonucleic acid (mRNA) expression in luteinized human granulosa cells in vitro. J Clin Endocrinol Metab. 1993; 77(6):1723–5.

37. Neulen J, Yan Z, Raczek S, Weindel K, Keck C, Weich HA et al. Human chorionic gonadotropin-dependent expression of vascular endothelial growth factor/vascular permeability factor in human granulosa cells: Importance in ovarian hyperstimulation syndrome. J Clin Endocrinol Metab. 1995; 80(6):1967–71.

38. Basu S, Nagy JA, Pal S, Vasile E, Eckelhoefer IA, Bliss VS et al. The neurotransmitter dopamine inhibits angiogenesis induced by vascular permeability factor/vascular endothelial growth factor. Nat Med. 2001; 7(5):569–74.

39. Gomez R, Simon C, Remohi J, Pellicer A. Vascular endothelial growth factor receptor-2 activation induces vascular permeability in hyperstimulated rats, and this effect is prevented by receptor blockade. Endocrinology. 143(11):4339–48.

40. Soares SR. Etiology of OHSS and use of dopamine agonists. Fertil Steril. 97(3):517–22.

41. Baumgarten M, Polanski L, Campbell B, Raine-Fenning N. Do dopamine agonists prevent or reduce the severity of ovarian hyperstimulation syndrome in women undergoing assisted reproduction? A systematic review and meta-analysis. Hum Fertil (Camb). 2013; 16(3):168–74.

25

Complications of Ovarian Stimulation: Multiple Pregnancies

Diane De Neubourg

Introduction

Ovarian stimulation (OS) is a common part of fertility treatments all over the world, and drugs, such as clomiphene citrate and gonadotropins, are widely used. These drugs all have their particular pharmacological mode of action, their proper indication, their cost, and pregnancy and live birth rates. However, multiple pregnancies are a well-known complication of ovarian stimulation, and the awareness has increased that these should be accounted for as complications of the therapy rather than as unpreventable side effects, particularly when high-order multiple pregnancies are considered.

A clear distinction should be made between controlled ovarian stimulation (COS) and ovarian stimulation in cases of ovulation disorders in which monofollicular growth is aimed for and which is called ovulation induction (OI). However, although monofollicular growth is the aim, the previous chapters have shown that this is not always easy to achieve in some groups of patients, such as patients with polycystic ovary syndrome (PCOS).

Controlled ovarian stimulation may be used in cases of unexplained infertility, minimal to mild endometriosis, or male subfertility often in combination with intrauterine insemination (IUI) in which an increasing amount of follicles should increase the chance of achieving a pregnancy. With COS, normoovulatory women are usually involved, and thus even a mild dose of ovarian stimulation may lead to multifollicular growth. In this group of patients, the increase in pregnancy rates should be balanced against the increase in risk of multiple pregnancies.

There are no data on outcomes from COS cycles without IUI in the literature, so reports from IUI cycles—although not entirely comparable—could give an estimate of both risk factors and the incidence of multiple pregnancies. The European IVF Monitoring (1) reported 9.3% twin deliveries and 0.5% triplets in 2009 in women <40 years treated with IUI using their husband's sperm. In 2005, COS with IUI and COS alone contributed as much as 22.8% to the national multiple birth cohort in the United States (2).

Studies on the factors that influence pregnancy rates are mostly reviews of retrospective studies and are descriptive in nature. Analysis of an important number of cycles may help to define risk factors for multiple pregnancies. However, interventions, such as cancellation of the cycle, aspiration of supernumerary follicles, escape IVF in case of unacceptable number of follicles, or selective reduction of a multifetal pregnancy, cannot be studied appropriately in retrospective cohorts.

In women treated by ovarian stimulation for OI or COS, both the pregnancy rates and also the risk of achieving a (high-order) multiple pregnancy should be considered. Therefore, appropriate ovarian stimulation should be a balance between these two outcome variables with a focus on completely preventing higher order multiple pregnancies and reducing the twin pregnancy rate to the lowest level possible.

Ovulation Induction

As previously mentioned, ovulation induction is the pharmacological treatment with clomiphene citrate, aromatase inhibitors, or gonadotropins and others (see previous chapters) to induce ovulation in a patient suffering from oligomenorrhea or anovulation.

For clomiphene citrate (CC), it is advised to start with the lowest dose of 50 mg daily for 5 days and to increase with 50 mg/day in the subsequent cycle if ovulation did not occur. This was analyzed in 259 normogonadotropic anovulatory patients for whom the cumulative live birth rate over 12 cycles was 41% with a multiple birth rate of 2% (3).

Although the use of CC is common and the availability of ultrasound monitoring is present in large parts of the world, there still is no evidence regarding the value of ultrasound (US) monitoring during CC treatment to reduce multiple pregnancy rates. A systematic review of all studies investigating the effects of US in the treatment of ovulatory dysfunction with CC showed insufficient evidence to suggest that ultrasound monitoring reduces multiple pregnancy rates or improves pregnancy rates (4). On the other hand, no indication that treatment with CC is safe without ultrasound monitoring was identified. The small number of relevant studies and the heterogeneity observed in the methodologies of each study prohibit reliable conclusions to be drawn. The NICE guideline of 2013 (5) advises that, for women who are taking CC, ultrasound monitoring should be offered during at least the first cycle to ensure that patients are taking a dose that minimizes the risk for multiple pregnancies. To summarize, no reliable conclusions can be drawn regarding the value of ultrasound monitoring in OI cycles to prevent multiple pregnancies because of the small number of relevant studies and the heterogeneity in the methodology of each study (LOE C).

In case of CC resistance or CC failure, gonadotropins can be used for OI. A retrospective cohort study of 748 patients in 2179 initiated cycles used a low-dose step-up protocol for OI. When three or more follicles of ≥16 mm were detected on ultrasound, the cycle was cancelled, and it was advised not to have unprotected intercourse. This strategy led to a cancellation rate of 22% of all cycles and to a pregnancy rate of 20% in the completed cycles. The multiple pregnancy rate was 11% (6).

For PCOS patients, aromatase inhibitors, such as letrozole, have been compared to CC for ovulation induction. A meta-analysis demonstrated that letrozole improved ovulation rates per patient but did not show differences in live birth nor multiple pregnancy rates (7) (LOE 1). A recent multicenter randomized trial comparing letrozole to clomiphene in PCOS patients did show a significant higher cumulative ovulation rate and more cumulative live births but did not find any differences in twin pregnancy. There were more major congenital anomalies with letrozole although this did not reach significance (8). However, this issue needs further follow up in larger series.

Controlled Ovarian Stimulation with or without IUI

Although COS with or without IUI is a different treatment option compared with OI, and also different patient populations are subjected to these treatments, lessons might be learned from COS to prevent multiple pregnancies in OI. Therefore, a short summary of evidence is provided here.

Identification of Risk Factors

A meta-analysis on the influence of the number of follicles on (multiple) pregnancy rates after COS in IUI programs performed by van Rumste et al. in 2008 (9) included 14 studies reporting on 11,599 cycles; only two studies were randomized controlled trials in contrast to 12 observational studies. The absolute pregnancy rate was 8.4% for monofollicular and 15% for multifollicular growth. The pooled odds ratio (OR) for pregnancy after two follicles as compared to one follicle was 1.6 (99% confidence interval [CI] 1.3–2.0) whereas for three and four follicles the pooled OR was 2.0 (99% CI 1.6–2.5) and 2.0 (95% CI 1.5–2.7), respectively. Compared with monofollicular growth, pregnancy rates increased by 5%, 8%, and 8% when stimulating two, three, and four follicles, respectively. The pooled OR for multiple pregnancies after two follicles was 1.7 (99% CI 0.8–3.6) and increased to 2.8 and 2.3 for three and four follicles, respectively. The risk of multiple pregnancies after two, three, and four follicles increased by 6%, 14%, and 10%. The absolute rate of multiple pregnancies was 0.3% after monofollicular and 2.8% after multifollicular growth. It was concluded that multifollicular growth is associated with increased pregnancy rates in IUI with COS (9) and that one should not aim for more than two follicles because in cycles with three or four follicles the multiple pregnancy rate increased without substantial gain in overall pregnancy rate.

Recently, identification of risk factors for multiple pregnancies has been done on the basis of 3375 gonadotropin-stimulated cycles in 1438 patients (10). Regression analysis revealed that the presence of at least two follicles ≥13 mm at ovulation trigger significantly increased clinical pregnancy rates (OR, 95% CI = 1.45, 1.18–1.78) and multiple pregnancy rates (MPR) (OR, 95% CI = 5.17, 2.16–12.41) and that an estradiol level >400 pg/ml significantly increased MPR (OR, 95% CI = 9.54, 2.31–39.42). A significant decrease in pregnancy rate was observed as age increases beyond 40 years (OR, 95% CI = 0.58, 0.44–0.76), but an association with multiple pregnancy rates could not be observed (10). On the basis of these and other patient-specific and cycle-specific variables, an applet has been developed to calculate the patient's chance to achieve a pregnancy and risk to develop a multiple pregnancy. However, one should bear in mind that risk estimates are insufficient in a patient population with an absolute contraindication for multiple pregnancies. In the general infertility population, two follicles and the risk of twin pregnancy may be acceptable after careful patient counseling.

Analysis of the Risks of Different Stimulation Protocols for Multiple Pregnancies

In a narrative review, McClamrock et al. (2) compared reproductive outcome after COS with clomiphene citrate, low-dose gonadotropins (≤75 IU), and high-dose gonadotropins (≥150 IU) in combination with IUI. They retrieved data from randomized controlled trials on the different stimulation protocols and analyzed them accordingly but without formal meta-analysis (Table 25.3). The authors (2) concluded first that an increasingly compelling case could be made in support of low-dose (≤75 IU) gonadotropin regimens for which per-cycle pregnancy rates of 8.7%–16.3% and absent high-order gestation have been noted in prospective randomized trials although a more mixed record was noted for the twin gestation category. A second conclusion (2) was that a strong case could also be made for clomiphene for which per-cycle pregnancy rates of 2.0%–19.3% have been noted in prospective randomized trials with virtual absence of high-order gestation and twin gestation rates ranging between 0% and 12.5%. However, these conclusions should be interpreted cautiously because they are based on a nonsystematic narrative review of the literature (2) without accounting for many forms of bias.

In a more thorough systematic Cochrane review (11) on the influence of the type of ovarian stimulation combined with IUI it was concluded that COS using gonadotropins increases pregnancy rates compared with the use of anti-estrogens (OR = 1.8, 95% CI 1.2–1.7). For studies that could be included in the comparison (11), there appeared to be no difference in the multiple pregnancy rates after COS with gonadotropins or anti-estrogens when calculated per patient (OR = 0.53; 95% CI 0.15–1.86) or per pregnancy (OR = 0.96; 95% CI 0.28–3.28). Doubling the starting dose of gonadotrophins did not increase pregnancy rates significantly (OR = 1.2; 95% CI 0.67–1.9) or affect multiple pregnancy rates (OR =

TABLE 25.3

Pregnancy and Multiple Pregnancy Rates with Clomiphene Citrate and Gonadotrophins Combined with IUI, according to Narrative Review (2)

Treatment	Number of Cycles	Pregnancy Rate per Cycle (%)	Twin Intrauterine Pregnancy Rate (%)	High-Order Intrauterine Pregnancy Rate (%)
Clomiphene citrate	3214	2–19.3	0–12.5	0–3.7
Low-dose gonadotrophins (≤75 IU)	1123	8.7–16.3	0–29.3	0
High-dose gonadotrophins (≥150 IU)	2227	8.7–19.2	0–28.6	0–9.3

3.11; 95% CI 0.48–20.13). Based on this systematic review, COS with gonadotropins is superior to COS with anti-estrogens in an IUI program without concomitant increased risk in multiple pregnancy rate. Nevertheless, it should be kept in mind that the risk for multiple pregnancy is more dependent on the number of stimulated follicles than on the type of product used for COS (gonadotropins or clomiphene citrate) as reviewed above in the section "Identification of risk factors."

Secondary Preventive Measures

Cancellation of the Cycle

When multifollicular development occurs during OI or COS a risk for (high-order) multiple pregnancies exists. As mentioned previously, on the basis of risk analysis by van Rumste et al. (9), one should aim for a maximum of two follicles in order to avoid high-order multiple pregnancies. Apart from common sense, there are no studies available in which risks of the number of follicles and their size are weighed and evaluated. There is a lack of evidence-based guidelines.

Aspiration of Supernumerary Follicles

Instead of cancellation of the cycle, supernumerary follicles can be aspirated vaginally under ultrasound guidance. In the studies reported, follicular aspiration was performed on the day of hCG administration when four or more follicles ≥14 mm were present. Three studies reported pregnancy rates and multiple pregnancy rates of 25%–27% and 0%–10%, respectively (2). However, patients should be counseled about this "invasive" option before they start with an OI or COS program.

Escape IVF

When many follicles have to be aspirated, it is important to discuss the possibility of a full oocyte aspiration performed as part of an ART treatment. This rescue procedure can certainly increase the chance of achieving a pregnancy with minimal risks for multiple pregnancies provided single embryo transfer is performed. However, the costs associated with ART are much higher than those associated with OI or COS. Furthermore, success of ART treatment can be compromised if oocytes ovulate prematurely, a common problem as most patients are not treated with a GnRH analogue or antagonist in the context of OI or COS. In principle, a GnRH antagonist can be added, but this is not always possible because follicle size usually exceeds 14 mm at the time of the decision to switch from OI or COS to IVF.

Selective Reduction of a Multi-Fetal Pregnancy

High-order multiple pregnancies will be at increased risk for adverse maternal and perinatal outcome. The balance between reducing the number of fetuses in an attempt to decrease maternal and perinatal risks versus continuation of the pregnancy has to be made individually based on patient counseling provided by ultrasound interventionalists, subspecialists in fetal-maternal medicine, neonatologists, and psychologists.

Conclusions

Ovulation induction aims at monofollicular growth. As pregnancy is more likely to occur with two follicles than with one, the risk for multiple pregnancies increases with 6% when two follicles are present instead of one. The risk for multiple pregnancies is independent of the drugs used, but it is recommended to use low-dose gonadotrophins with gonadotrophin stimulation. In case more than two follicles develop, secondary preventive measures should be considered.

TABLE 25.1

Level of Evidence of Statements

Statement	Level of Evidence
Pregnancy is more likely to occur with two follicles than with one in COS cycles (9).	1a
The risk of multiple pregnancies for two follicles as compared to one follicle increases by 6% (9).	1a
There is no difference in the risk of multiple pregnancies between anti-estrogens and gonadotropins in IUI programs (11).	1a

TABLE 25.2

Grade of Strength for Recommendations

Recommendation	Grade Strength
Low-dose gonadotropins should be used instead of high-dose gonadotropins.	A
COS should aim for no more than two follicles.	B
Follicle aspiration may prevent multiple pregnancies while maintaining acceptable pregnancy rates.	C
In case of multifollicular development, escape ART (conversion from IUI into ART) can prevent multiple pregnancies while maintaining acceptable pregnancy rates when combined with single embryo transfer.	C

REFERENCES

1. Kupka MS, Ferraretti AP, de Mouzon J, Erb K, D'Hooghe T, Castilla JA, Calhaz-Jorge C et al. Assisted reproductive technology in Europe, 2010: Results generated from European registers by ESHRE. Hum Reprod. 2014; 29:2099–113.
2. McClamrock HD, Jones HW Jr, Adashi EY. Ovarian stimulation and intrauterine insemination at the quarter centennial: Implications for the multiple births epidemic. Fertil Steril. 2012; 4:802–9.
3. van Santbrink EJ, Eijkemans MJ, Laven JS, Fauser BC. Patient-tailored conventional ovulation induction algorithms in anovulatory infertility. Trends Endocrinol Metab. 2005; 16:381–9.
4. Galazis N, Zertalis M, Haoula Z, Atiomo W. Is ultrasound monitoring of the ovaries during ovulation induction by clomiphene citrate essential? A systematic review. J Obstet Gynaecol. 2011; 31:566–71.
5. National Institute for Health and Clinical excellence. Assessment and treatment for people with fertility problems. NICE clinical guideline 156, February 2013.
6. Wang JX, Kwan M, Davies MJ, Kirby C, Judd S, Norman RJ. Risk of multiple pregnancy when infertility is treated with ovulation induction by gonadotropins. Fertil Steril. 2003; 80:664–5.
7. Misso ML, Wong JL, Teede HJ, Hart R, Rombauts L, Melder AM et al. Aromatase inhibitors for PCOS: A systematic review and meta-analysis. Hum Reprod Update. 2012; 18:301–12.
8. Legro RS, Brzyski RG, Diamond MP, Coutifaris C, Schlaff WD, Casson P et al. Letrozole versus clomiphene for infertility in the polycystic ovary syndrome. N Engl J Med. 2014; 371:119–29.
9. van Rumste MM, Custers IM, van der Veen F, van Wely M, Evers JL, Mol BW. The influence of the number of follicles on pregnancy rates in intrauterine insemination with ovarian stimulation: A meta-analysis. Hum Reprod Update 2008; 6:563–70.
10. Goldman RH, Batsis M, Petrozza JC, Souter I. Patient-specific predictions of outcome after gonadotropin ovulation induction/intrauterine insemination. Fertil Steril. 2014; 101:1649–55.
11. Cantineau AE, Cohlen BJ. Ovarian stimulation protocols (anti-oestrogens, gonadotrophins with and without agonists/antagonists) for intrauterine insemenation (IUI) in women with subfertility. Cochrane Database Syst Rev 2007; 2:CD005356.

26

Long-Term Complications of Anovulation

Joop S. E. Laven

Introduction

Anovulation, especially if untreated, is associated with several short-, middle long-, and long-term health sequelae. WHO 1 and WHO 3 anovulatory states are characterized by hyopogonadism, and therefore, they cause hypo-estrogenism. Long-lasting underexposure to estrogens may lead, in these circumstances, to osteoporosis (i.e., decreased bone mineral density [BMD]), mood and cognitive disturbances, and sexual dysfunction as well as accelerated cardiovascular aging and subsequent cardiovascular disease and, if left untreated, a reduced life span. Similarly, since WHO 2 anovulation and especially PCOS are associated with obesity, insulin resistance, and metabolic syndrome, these women also have an increased risk of develop type 2 diabetes, hypertension, and probably cardiovascular disease.

WHO 1 Hypogonadotropic Hypogonadism (HH)

Functional hypothalamic amenorrhea is related to profound impairment of reproductive functions, including anovulation and infertility. Women's health, in this disorder, is disturbed in several aspects, including the skeletal system, cardiovascular system, and mental problems. Patients manifest a decrease in bone mass density, which is related to an increase in fracture risk. Therefore, osteopenia and osteoporosis are the main long-term complications of HH. Cardiovascular complications include endothelial dysfunction and abnormal changes in the lipid profile. HH patients present significantly higher depression and anxiety and also sexual problems compared to healthy subjects (1).

Patients with HH are threatened by a low peak bone mass (PBM) not only due to hypo-estrogenism. Other important factors include improper diet (low calcium and vitamin D3 intake), undernutrition, and excessive exercise. Moreover, HH individuals had a decreased fat tissue mass and an imbalanced relationship between body weight, fat tissue mass, and lean body mass. More attention should be paid to exercise among women. For most of the young women, exercise causes a positive effect, improving health and physical fitness. However, excessive exercise (exercise-related hypothalamic amenorrhea) does not improve BMD but leads to osteopenia. Abnormally low BMD and osteoporosis in exercising women relate to premature bone loss and micro-architectural deterioration (1).

Several investigators have demonstrated a correlation between HH and endothelial dysfunction. The Women's Ischemia Syndrome Evaluation (WISE) study found a significant association between premenopausal angiographic coronary artery disease and hypothalamic hypogonadism. Impaired cardiovascular function in hypothalamic amenorrhea is believed to be linked mainly to hypo-estrogenism, but it is also aggravated by negative energy balance and metabolic disturbances. Patients with HH are characterized by an impaired lipid profile and are at risk of glucose metabolism abnormalities. However, the influence of hypo-estrogenism in young women with HH on cardiovascular health requires further studies. Especially the issue of the long-term consequences of HH on CVD risk needs to be cleared to possibly minimize the risk of cardiovascular events in this group of women (1).

Women with HH endorsed more dysfunctional attitudes, had greater difficulty in coping with daily stresses, and tended to endorse greater interpersonal dependence than eumenorrheic women. WHO 1 patients present a particular susceptibility to common life events, restrictive disordered eating, depressive traits, and psychosomatic disorders. Psychological problems are aggravated by the fact that HH is associated with anxiety, depressive symptoms, and high rates of mood disorders. The mediating effects of anxiety and depression may explain the occurrence of sexual dysfunction, which is potentially associated with WHO 1 anovulation. Finally, the hormonal background of sexual dysfunction in FHA may be related to profound hypo-estrogenism and hypoandrogenemia (1).

WHO 2 Normogonadotropic Normo-Estrogenic Anovulation (PCOS)

Women with PCOS are more likely to have upper body fat distribution compared with weight-matched controls. Greater abdominal or visceral adiposity is associated with greater insulin resistance, which could exacerbate the reproductive and metabolic abnormalities in PCOS (2). It is known that obesity is associated with PCOS, but its causal role in this condition has yet to be determined. Very few studies report the association of BMI with menstrual irregularity. Few randomized controlled studies have been performed on lifestyle interventions, but these suggest substantial reproductive and metabolic benefits (3,4).

Insulin resistance is a prevalent finding in women with PCOS. It is most prevalent and severe in those with the classic phenotype, involving hyperandrogenism and chronic anovulation. Women with PCOS assessed by the Rotterdam criteria yet with regular cycles are metabolically less abnormal. The cellular and molecular mechanisms of insulin resistance in PCOS differ from those in other common insulin-resistant states, such as obesity and type 2 diabetes. In vivo insulin action is profoundly decreased in skeletal muscle secondary to signaling defects, but hepatic insulin resistance is present only in obese women with PCOS. There is a synergistic negative effect of having both PCOS and obesity on insulin action. Pancreatic beta-cell dysfunction is also present in PCOS but may be more related to type 2 diabetes risk factors as this dysfunction is most severe in women with a first-degree relative who has type 2 diabetes. Extensive evidence indicates that hyperinsulinemia contributes directly to reproductive dysfunction in PCOS. Women with the classic hyperandrogenic PCOS phenotype have significantly increased rates of the metabolic syndrome compared with reproductively normal women of similar age and weight (2).

Insulin resistance is a prominent feature of PCOS. There is now compelling evidence from epidemiologic data that PCOS is associated with increased risk of impaired glucose tolerance, gestational diabetes, and type 2 diabetes. Screening making use of an oral glucose tolerance test is indicated in obese women with PCOS and/or those with increased visceral adiposity as measured by waist circumference. Risk of impaired glucose metabolism or diabetes is highest in women who have both oligo-ovulation or anovulation and hyperandrogenism, and the risk is further amplified by obesity. Management of women at risk for type 2 diabetes should include diet and lifestyle improvement as the first-line treatment. Metformin treatment is indicated in those with impaired glucose metabolism who do not respond adequately to calorie restriction and lifestyle changes. In those with frank diabetes, metformin is safe and effective whereas there is concern about the use of thiazolidinediones and glucagonlike peptide-1 analogues in women of reproductive age (2).

PCOS at any age is characterized by greater odds for elevated CVD risk markers. Elevated markers occur without obesity and are magnified with obesity. Dyslipidemia, impaired glucose tolerance as well as type 2 diabetes (classic risk indicators of atherosclerosis and CVD) are more prevalent in women with PCOS even when weight matched with normal control women. Dyslipidemia reflected by altered levels of triglycerides, HDL, LDL, and non-HDL is prevalent in women with PCOS and is more severe in hyperandrogenic women. Non-HDL cholesterol and waist measurement appear to be the best clinical indicators of elevated CVD risk. All markers reflect a greater magnitude of risk when women are diagnosed into the hyperandrogenic phenotypes compared to the non-hyperandrogenic phenotype (2).

Although most of the surrogate markers do predict a higher CVD risk in women with PCOS, there is only very limited data available on the real hard clinical end points, that is, stroke and coronary heart disease and myocardial infarction. In fact, there are only two long-term follow-up studies indicating women with polycystic ovary syndrome do not have markedly higher than average mortality from circulatory disease even though the condition is strongly associated with diabetes, lipid abnormalities, and other cardiovascular risk factors (5,6).

There are some data to support that women with PCOS have a two- to threefold increased risk for endometrial cancer. Most endometrial cancers are well differentiated and have a good prognosis. Limited data exist that do support the conclusion that women with PCOS are not at increased risk for ovarian cancer. Similarly, there are no data to support the fact that women with PCOS are at greater risk to develop breast cancer (2).

Patients with PCOS are at risk for psychological and behavioral disorders and reduced quality of life (QOL). Studies in this area have been hampered by the existence of only one validated disease-specific questionnaire, the QOL Questionnaire for Women with PCOS (PCOSQ). A review of generic and specific QOL studies in women with PCOS concluded that PCOS had a significant detrimental effect on QOL compared to women without PCOS. Moreover, weight issues are most apt to affect QOL. However, from other validated measures, it appears that patients with PCOS are at higher risk for developing significant psychological difficulties, such as depression and anxiety, compared with healthy controls. Finally, women suffering from PCOS may also be at risk for eating disorders and sexual and relational dysfunction although this evidence is inconsistent (7).

WHO 3 Anovulation or POI

Early menopause has been associated with increased cardiovascular disease (CVD), but the causal nature of the relationship has been unclear. For a comprehensive review, see Santoro (8). It has been hypothesized that women with preexisting CVD are more likely to undergo early menopause. However, there are also epidemiological data to suggest that early menopause is an independent risk factor for CVD (9,10). Moreover, there are data to suggest that CVD is more severe in women with early menopause. In a recent prospective study of a myocardial infarction registry, women with early menopause are at higher risk of angina after myocardial infarction (MI), independent of comorbidities, severity and quality of care (11). Notably, in this study, women with menopause before the age of 40 years were more likely to be smokers, but they did not have other additional comorbidities that differed from the age-appropriate menopause group (11). Women undergoing premenopausal bilateral oophorectomy and not treated with estrogen had a near doubling of cardiovascular mortality in a cohort followed in Olmsted County, Minnesota (12). Moreover, bilateral oophorectomy performed before age 45 years is associated with increased mortality for neurological or mental diseases (13).

By comparing women with POI with women who experienced natural menopause with respect to CVD risk factors, it has been shown that several CVD risk factors are related to estrogen deprivation. Aging does not have an important impact on CVD within the age range of this study group (14). Longitudinal studies have demonstrated an 80% increased risk of mortality from ischemic heart disease in POI compared with those with menopause at 49–55 years. This risk is more pronounced in those who have never used estrogens. The increased risk of CVD may be due to direct effects on the endothelium or through alterations to traditional cardiovascular risk factors such as adverse effects on lipid profile, reduced insulin sensitivity, and metabolic syndrome (8).

Sexual dysfunction is a common problem among women with POI with decreased sexual well being, arousal, frequency, and increased dyspareunia. Sexual dysfunction is more complex the younger the age at diagnosis, and it is also affected by etiology, parity, premorbid personality, and the partner's response. Management includes psychosexual counseling and HRT. Women with POI have lower androgen levels compared to healthy controls, and consideration should be given to androgen replacement. However, there are only limited data investigating the role of androgen replacement in POI, and no studies have explored its effect on sexual function (8).

An increased risk of cognitive impairment is also observed in POI. In a French, population-based cohort, POI was associated with negative effects on cognitive function in later life, including increased risk of poor verbal fluency and impaired visual memory. There was no clear evidence that use of HRT reduced the risk of cognitive decline, but HRT use was self-reported at the age of at least 65 years, and therefore, recall bias may have affected the results (15).

Women with POI have significantly lower BMD as well as an increased fracture risk. There is now evidence to suggest that HRT seems to preserve BMD and, moreover, can actually restore BMD to levels comparable to control groups. Finally, the use of HRT in case it is used for at least 3 years may reduce fracture risk (8).

In most women, earlier reproductive aging seems to be detrimental to overall health and even life expectancy. Life expectancy in POI is about 2 years less than those who have menopause over 55 years, and this is thought to be due to an excess of deaths due to CVD, osteoporosis, and neurocognitive

TABLE 26.1

Level of Evidence of Statements

Statement	Level of Evidence
Long-lasting underexposure to estrogens may lead, in these circumstances, to osteoporosis (i.e., decreased bone mineral density [BMD]), mood and cognitive disturbances, and sexual dysfunction as well as accelerated cardiovascular aging and subsequent cardiovascular disease and, if left untreated, a reduced life span.	2
WHO 2 anovulation and especially PCOS are associated with obesity, insulin resistance, and metabolic syndrome; these women also have an increased risk to develop type 2 diabetes, hypertension, and probably cardiovascular disease.	2
WHO 1 anovulation is associated with osteopenia, osteoporosis, endothelial dysfunction, and dyslipidemia compared to healthy ovulatory women.	2
Women with HH present with significantly higher depression and anxiety and also sexual problems compared to healthy subjects.	2
HH women have lowered PBM because of their hypo-estrogenic state along with other factors, such as low calcium and vitamin D3 intake, undernutrition, and excessive exercise.	2
HH is associated with significant coronary artery disease and endothelial dysfunction.	2
WHO 1 patients present a particular susceptibility to common life events, restrictive disordered eating, depressive traits, and psychosomatic disorders.	2
Increased adiposity, particularly abdominal, is associated with HA and increased metabolic risk.	
Women with PCOS are at an increased risk for developing impaired glucose tolerance and type 2 diabetes.	2
Weight loss is likely beneficial for both reproductive and metabolic dysfunction in this setting. Weight loss is likely insufficient as a treatment for PCOS in normal-weight women.	2
Women with PCOS suffer more often from psychological and behavioral disorders and reduced quality of life.	2
Women with PCOS share many of the risk factors associated with the development of endometrial cancer, including obesity, hyperinsulinism, type 2 diabetes, and abnormal uterine bleeding. Hence, they do have an increased lifelong risk for developing endometrial cancer.	2
Early menopause has been associated with increased CVD risk.	2
Women with early menopause are at higher risk of angina after myocardial infarction (MI), independent of comorbidities, severity and quality of care.	2
Bilateral oophorectomy leads to an increase in CVD as well as to an increase in neurological or mental diseases.	2
Women with POI experience more sexual dysfunction compared to healthy controls.	2
Women with POI are at risk for cognitive impairment.	2
Life expectancy in POI is about 2 years less than those who have menopause over 55 years, and this is thought to be due to an excess of deaths due to CVD, osteoporosis, and neurocognitive decline.	2
Nonhormonal therapies, such as SSRIs, serotonin and norepinephrine reuptake inhibitors, or gabapentin may have a role in the management of vasomotor symptoms in women who decline HRT or in whom HRT is contraindicated.	3
There is no evidence for the use of complementary or herbal preparations in POI.	2

decline (16). Whether this link is strictly a result of reproductive aging or a reflection of the effects of reproductive aging on other endocrine systems still requires more research. Clearly, reversing the effects of reproductive aging by counteracting hormone deficiencies to prevent long-term morbidity and mortality has not been a successful clinical approach. Likely, the general cardiovascular risk profile of individual women plays an important role in determining the baseline risk of adverse risks and the impact the differences in reproductive aging play in modifying risk (8).

General lifestyle and dietary measures to reduce risk of cardiovascular disease (CVD) and osteoporosis should be recommended. This includes adequate dietary intake or supplementation of calcium and vitamin D, regular weight-bearing exercise and reduction in smoking alcohol and caffeine. Nonhormonal therapies, such as selective serotonin reuptake inhibitors, serotonin and norepinephrine reuptake inhibitors, or gabapentin may have a role in the management of vasomotor symptoms in women who decline HRT or in whom HRT is contraindicated, but they will have no benefit on future risk of osteoporosis and CVD. There is no evidence for the use of complementary or herbal preparations in POI, and hormone replacement forms the mainstay of pharmacological management. Bisphosphonates are not recommended in women who wish to achieve pregnancy as they have a long half-life and fetal effects are unknown (8).

TABLE 26.2

Grade of Strength for Recommendations

Recommendation	Grade Strength
In WHO 1 HH women, more attention should be paid to exercise among women. For most of the young women, exercise causes a positive effect, improving health and physical fitness.	B
Especially the issue of the long-term consequences of HH on CVD risk needs to be cleared to possibly minimize the risk of cardiovascular events in this group of women.	C
Screening in adolescents and women with PCOS for increased adiposity, by BMI calculation and measurement of waist circumference, should be done routinely.	B
An oral glucose tolerance test (OGTT) (consisting of fasting and 2-hour glucose level using a 75-g oral glucose load) should be used to screen for impaired glucose tolerance (IGT) and T2DM in adolescents and adult women with PCOS.	B
Adolescents and women with PCOS should be screened for CVD risk factors, such as a family history of early CVD, cigarette smoking, IGT/T2DM, hypertension, dyslipidemia, obstructive sleep apnea, and obesity (especially increased abdominal adiposity).	B
Exercise therapy in the management of overweight and obesity in PCOS might be helpful.	C
Weight loss strategies should start with calorie-restricted diets (with no evidence that one type of diet is superior) for adolescents and women with PCOS who are overweight or obese.	C
The use of hormonal contraceptives (i.e., oral contraceptives, patch, or vaginal ring) as first-line management for menstrual abnormalities is recommended. Especially in case hirsutism or acne is part of PCOS, this approach treats both entities.	B
Screen women and adolescents with PCOS for depression and anxiety by history and, if identified, providing appropriate referral and/or treatment.	B
Routine ultrasound screening for endometrial thickness in women with PCOS should not be done.	B
Women with POI should be treated with HRT to reduce their complaints as well as their risk for CVD.	C
Women with POI and sexual dysfunction should be counseled by a sexologist and treated with HRT.	C
Women with cognitive impairment due to POI seem to benefit from HRT.	C
HRT has not been successful in reversing the effects of reproductive aging to prevent long-term morbidity and mortality.	B
General lifestyle and dietary measures to reduce risk of cardiovascular disease (CVD) and osteoporosis should be recommended.	B
Do not use bisphosphonates in women who are trying to establish a pregnancy.	B

REFERENCES

1. Meczekalski B, Katulski K, Czyzyk A, Podfigurna-Stopa A, Maciejewska-Jeske M. Functional hypothalamic amenorrhea and its influence on women's health. J Endocrinol Invest. 2014.
2. Fauser BC, Tarlatzis BC, Rebar RW, Legro RS, Balen AH, Lobo R et al. Consensus on women's health aspects of polycystic ovary syndrome (PCOS): The Amsterdam ESHRE/ASRM-Sponsored 3rd PCOS Consensus Workshop Group. Fertil Steril. 2012; 97(1):28–38 e25.
3. Moran LJ, Pasquali R, Teede HJ, Hoeger KM, Norman RJ. Treatment of obesity in polycystic ovary syndrome: A position statement of the Androgen Excess and Polycystic Ovary Syndrome Society. Fertil Steril. 2009; 92(6):1966–82.
4. Moran LJ, Misso ML, Wild RA, Norman RJ. Impaired glucose tolerance, type 2 diabetes and metabolic syndrome in polycystic ovary syndrome: A systematic review and meta-analysis. Hum Reprod Update. 2010; 16(4):347–63.
5. Pierpoint T, McKeigue PM, Isaacs AJ, Wild SH, Jacobs HS. Mortality of women with polycystic ovary syndrome at long-term follow-up. J Clin Epidemiol. 1998; 51(7):581–6.
6. Schmidt J, Landin-Wilhelmsen K, Brannstrom M, Dahlgren E. Cardiovascular disease and risk factors in PCOS women of postmenopausal age: A 21-year controlled follow-up study. J Clin Endocrinol Metab. 2011; 96(12):3794–803.
7. Himelein MJ, Thatcher SS. Polycystic ovary syndrome and mental health: A review. Obstet Gynecol Surv. 2006; 61(11):723–32.
8. Maclaran K, Panay N. Current concepts in premature ovarian insufficiency. Womens Health (Lond Engl). 2015; 11(2):169–82.
9. van der Schouw YT, van der Graaf Y, Steyerberg EW, Eijkemans JC, Banga JD. Age at menopause as a risk factor for cardiovascular mortality. Lancet. 1996; 347(9003):714–8.
10. Joakimsen O, Bonaa KH, Stensland-Bugge E, Jacobsen BK. Population-based study of age at menopause and ultrasound assessed carotid atherosclerosis: The Tromso Study. J Clin Epidemiol. 2000; 53(5):525–30.
11. Parashar S, Reid KJ, Spertus JA, Shaw LJ, Vaccarino V. Early menopause predicts angina after myocardial infarction. Menopause. 2010; 17(5):938–45.
12. Rivera CM, Grossardt BR, Rhodes DJ, Brown RD, Jr., Roger VL, Melton LJ, 3rd et al. Increased cardiovascular mortality after early bilateral oophorectomy. Menopause. 2009; 16(1):15–23.
13. Rivera CM, Grossardt BR, Rhodes DJ, Rocca WA. Increased mortality for neurological and mental diseases following early bilateral oophorectomy. Neuroepidemiology. 2009; 33(1):32–40.
14. Senoz S, Direm B, Gulekli B, Gokmen O. Estrogen deprivation, rather than age, is responsible for the poor lipid profile and carbohydrate metabolism in women. Maturitas. 1996; 25(2):107–14.
15. Ryan J, Scali J, Carriere I, Amieva H, Rouaud O, Berr C et al. Impact of a premature menopause on cognitive function in later life. BJOG. 2014; 121(13):1729–39.
16. Ossewaarde ME, Bots ML, Verbeek AL, Peeters PH, van der Graaf Y, Grobbee DE et al. Age at menopause, cause-specific mortality and total life expectancy. Epidemiology. 2005; 16(4):556–62.

27

Predicting Outcome of Treating Anovulation

Yvonne V. Louwers and Evert J. P. van Santbrink

Introduction

Treatment of anovulatory infertility aims at restoring normal ovarian physiology, that is, mono-follicular growth and mono-ovulation. First-line ovulation induction treatment with anti-estrogen clomiphene citrate (CC) has the advantage of a high response rate and low costs as well as minor side effects and complications. In case of clomiphene-resistant anovulation (CRA) or failure to conceive (CRF), second-line treatment to induce ovulation consists of daily administration of exogenous FSH. To enhance the ovarian sensitivity for FSH stimulation, laparoscopic electrocoagulation of the ovaries (LEO, Chapter 18) and the use of insulin sensitizers (i.e., Metformin, Chapter 17) are proposed. These modalities are utilized in patients after CRA and may be combined with the use of CC or FSH. Although effective, treatment with CC and FSH is complicated by the limited control of ovarian response due to large inter- and intrapatient variability. Development of prediction models taking into account individual patient characteristics may be a step forward in optimizing the decision-making process in the treatment of normogonadotropic anovulation, resulting in a more patient-tailored treatment.

Overview of Existing Evidence

Clomiphene Citrate

Over the last decades, several prediction models for success with ovulation induction have been proposed. In general, these prediction models used clinically easily accessible parameters.

In a prospective longitudinal single-center study, Imani et al. developed a model to predict the individual chances of live birth after CC administration using two distinct prediction models combined in a normogram. Univariate and multivariate analyses were used to identify these predictors. In this study population, a cumulative conception rate of 73% was reached within nine CC-induced ovulatory cycles. Body mass index and hyperandrogenemia were observed to be the predominant predictors for ovulation after CC treatment whereas age and cycle history dictated pregnancy chances in ovulatory women (1). These conclusions have been largely confirmed about 10 years later in an independent study population (2).

FSH

In addition, similar models have been considered for FSH low-dose ovulation induction. Age, duration of infertility, and insulin/glucose ratio were combined to predict live birth rate in clomiphene-resistant anovulatory women receiving FSH treatment (3). In this study, clomiphene-resistant anovulatory women receiving FSH achieved a cumulative 2-year live birth rate of 71%. Cox regression was used for univariate and multivariate analysis relating initial screening characteristics to the cumulative pregnancy rate, leading to singleton live birth. Subsequently, the latter prediction model was validated in an independent cohort of patients with polycystic ovary syndrome (4). Veltman et al. also included BMI resulting in a better predictive index of live birth: 60% at 12 months and 78% at 24 months.

Insulin Sensitizers (See Also Chapter 17)

The presumed central role of insulin resistance in hyperandrogenism in PCOS is the reason that insulin sensitizers were introduced in ovulation induction. By lowering insulin resistance, ovarian dysfunction may diminish and ovarian responsiveness to FSH improve. This effect might be more evident in overweight (BMI > 28) and insulin-resistant PCOS patients. Clinically, Metformin is proving to be effective as an adjuvant to CC in CRA patients. In only a few small studies, it is suggested that Metformin cotreatment in gonadotropin induction of ovulation results in a decreased amount of FSH needed, a significantly shorter stimulation period, and more monofollicular cycles.

Laparoscopic Electrocautery of the Ovaries (LEO) or Laparoscopic Drilling of the Ovaries (LOD, See Also Chapter 18)

Patient characteristics reported to predict chances for ovulation and pregnancy after LEO in a WHO 2 infertility population, failing to ovulate or conceive after CC treatment, were hyperandrogenism (T and FAI) and BMI whereas elevated LH serum levels increased chances for pregnancy (5). These data could not be confirmed by a smaller prospective study in a group of patients with CRA (6). Only age at menarche and LH/FSH ratio were significantly related to treatment response.

Genetic Factors

Also in the field of pharmacogenetics, efforts have been made to identify genetic factors that influence the outcome of ovulation induction treatment. PCOS patients carrying the Ser680 allele in the *follicle stimulating hormone receptor* gene were more often clomiphene citrate–resistant than noncarriers (7). Furthermore, genetic variants in the STK11 gene seem associated with ovulation induction outcome in PCOS (8).

Discussion

Interestingly, following CC treatment, approximately 70%–80% of the women gained ovulations whereas only 40%–50% of them will conceive. Different predictive parameters are likely underlying this large discrepancy between successful regaining ovulations and actual pregnancy rate, insinuating that anovulatory is a complex multifactorial phenomenon. Taking this into account, it seems obvious that one treatment regimen will be not be suitable for all patients' anovulatory subfertility. Current prediction models for ovulation induction outcome have been developed in single center prospective follow-up studies. Large multicenter randomized controlled trials are lacking in identifying predictors of ovulation induction outcome. The performance of these prediction models is often evaluated with a receiver operating characteristic (ROC) curve. As a measure of model performance, usually the area under the ROC curve (AUC), also known as c-statistic, is used. However, in the field of reproductive medicine, the value for this c-statistic is low because it only expresses discrimination and is, as such, not a good measure of the extent to which predictive models can be used in clinical practice (9). Therefore, we need to realize that in reproductive medicine, prognostic models that perfectly predict pregnancy in anovulatory subfertility most likely do not exist. However, this does not mean that these prediction models can be supportive in terms of clinical decision making (see further Table 27.3).

Conclusions

Body mass index and hyperandrogenemia seem to be the predominant predictors for ovulation after CC treatment whereas age and cycle history dictate pregnancy chances in ovulatory women. Apart from

TABLE 27.3

Predictors for Success (+) or Failure (–) of Ovulation Induction Treatment

	CC	Metformin	LEO
Age ≥ 28 years		+ (10)	
Duration of subfertility	– (2)	– (2)	– (5/2011)
Oligo-amenorrhea	O (2)		
BMI	– (2)	+ (10,2,11,12)	– (5/2011)
Insulin resistance/hyperandrogenism	– (2)	+ (10)	– (5/2011)
Ovarian volume	– (2)		

TABLE 27.1

Level of Evidence of Statements

Statement	Level of Evidence
Body mass index and hyperandrogenemia seem the predominant predictors for ovulation after CC treatment.	2a
Age and cycle history seem the predominant predictors pregnancy rate after CC treatment.	2a
Metformin might be effective as an adjuvant to CC in CRA patients.	2a
Patients with hyperandrogenism (T and FAI) and elevated BMI had decreased chances of conceive after LEO.	2a
Presence of the FSH receptor polymorphism might predict clomiphene resistance.	2a

TABLE 27.2

Grade of Strength for Recommendations

Recommendation	Grade Strength
Body mass index and hyperandrogenemia seem the predominant predictors for ovulation induction outcome.	B
Individual patient characteristics should be taken into account.	D
Prognostic models can be supportive in terms of clinical decision making.	D

these clinical and endocrine parameters, the genetically determined sensitivity of the FSH receptor might be an important factor too in predicting treatment outcome. This implies that genetic data might have a role in further optimizing the existing patient-tailored strategies in ovulation induction treatment in anovulatory women. Obviously, it is a major challenge to combine clinical, endocrine, and genetic factors to reliably predict outcome of ovulation induction and, even more importantly, healthy live birth.

REFERENCES

1. Imani B, Eijkemans MJ, te Velde ER, Habbema JD, Fauser BC. A nomogram to predict the probability of live birth after clomiphene citrate induction of ovulation in normogonadotropic oligoamenorrheic infertility. Fertil Steril. 2002; 77:91–7.
2. Rausch ME, Legro RS, Barnhart HX, Schlaff WD, Carr BR, Diamond MP et al. Predictors of pregnancy in women with polycystic ovary syndrome. J Clin Endocrinol Metab. 2009; 94:3458–66.
3. Eijkemans MJ, Imani B, Mulders AG, Habbema JD, Fauser BC. High singleton live birth rate following classical ovulation induction in normogonadotrophic anovulatory infertility (WHO 2). Hum Reprod. 2003; 18:2357–62.
4. Veltman-Verhulst SM, Fauser BC, Eijkemans MJ. High singleton live birth rate confirmed after ovulation induction in women with anovulatory polycystic ovary syndrome: Validation of a prediction model for clinical practice. Fertil Steril. 2012; 98:761–8, e761.

5. Amer SA, Li TC, Ledger WL. Ovulation induction using laparoscopic ovarian drilling in women with polycystic ovarian syndrome: Predictors of success. Hum Reprod. 2004; 19:1719–24.

6. van Wely M, Bayram N, van der Veen F, Bossuyt PM. Predictors for treatment failure after laparoscopic electrocautery of the ovaries in women with clomiphene citrate resistant polycystic ovary syndrome. Hum Reprod. 2005; 20:900–5.

7. Simoni M, Tempfer CB, Destenaves B, Fauser BC. Functional genetic polymorphisms and female reproductive disorders: Part 1: Polycystic ovary syndrome and ovarian response. Hum Reprod Update. 2008; 14:459–84.

8. Legro RS, Barnhart HX, Schlaff WD, Carr BR, Diamond MP, Carson SA et al. Ovulatory response to treatment of polycystic ovary syndrome is associated with a polymorphism in the STK11 gene. J Clin Endocrinol Metab. 2008; 93:792–800.

9. Coppus SF, van der Veen F, Opmeer BC, Mol BW, Bossuyt PM. Evaluating prediction models in reproductive medicine. Hum Reprod. 2009; 24:1774–8.

10. Moll E, Korevaar JC, Bossuyt PM, van der Veen F. Does adding metformin to clomifene citrate lead to higher pregnancy rates in a subset of women with polycystic ovary syndrome? Hum Reprod. 2008; 23:1830–4

11. Palomba S, Orio F Jr, Nardo LG, Falbo A, Russo T, Corea D et al. Metformin administration versus laparoscopic ovarian diathermy in clomiphene citrate-resistant women with polycystic ovary syndrome: A prospective parallel randomized double-blind placebo-controlled trial. J Clin Endocrinol Metab. 2004; 89:4801–9.

12. Creanga AA, Bradley HM, McCormick C, Witkop CT. Use of metformin in polycystic ovary syndrome: A meta-analysis. Obstet Gynecol. 2008; 111:959–68.

28

Future Prospects

Renato Pasquali

Introduction

In the last two decades, major improvements in ovulation induction protocols and techniques, including assisted reproductive technologies (ARTs) have been achieved, leading to a steady rise in pregnancy rates as demonstrated by national statistics worldwide. Anovulatory infertility, particularly the type due to polycystic ovary syndrome (PCOS), represents one of the major factors responsible for the increasing resort to ovulation induction techniques worldwide (1). Because the increasing age of individuals with infertility problems represents a major concern, practitioners, gynecologists, and other specialists are faced with a rise in direct or indirect questions and problems about ovulation induction techniques.

Evaluation of Ovarian Reserve

The development of knowledge on the role of the anti-Müllerian hormone (AMH) in ovarian physiology and pathology has opened a new chance in the diagnostic workup of female infertility. The measurement of blood concentrations of AMH has been applied to a wide array of clinical conditions based on its ability to reflect the number of antral and pre-antral follicles in the ovaries. In addition, AMH blood levels may help in choosing the ovarian stimulation protocol and the dose of gonadotropins to begin with in order to limit the risks of ovarian hyperstimulation syndrome (OHSS) or cancellation of cycles due to poor ovarian response although this still represents a matter of further research. Despite all these premises, it should be noted that the evaluation of AMH has not yet been accepted as an alternative to ultrasonography in the diagnosis of PCOS nor in that of premature ovarian failure although it has been proved to be useful in daily practice. This is partly due to the fact that we ought to have a reliable assay to measure AMH whereas, at present, there is evidence that most assays are lacking in accuracy, precision, sensitivity, and reproducibility. AMH assays continue to evolve and technical issues remain. The absence of an international standard is a key issue, particularly in the area of infertility treatment (2).

Treatment with Gonadotropins

Ovarian stimulation with gonadotropins is considered a second-line treatment for the PCOS patients with infertility (3). At present, the use of gonadotropins and gonadotropin-releasing hormone (GnRH) analogues has allowed the tailoring, based on an individual basis, of several ovarian stimulation procedures. The two most commonly used gonadotropin forms are urinary human menopausal gonadotropin (hMG) and recombinant follicle stimulating hormone (FSH) in combination with gonadotropin-releasing hormone (GnRH) agonists or antagonists. Several studies have shown that gonadotropins may be effective after an ovarian stimulation with clomiphene citrate (CC) in patients with CC resistance; however, approximately two thirds of patients may positively respond in term of live birth rates (4). Recently, low-dose FSH treatment has been found to be superior to CC as first-line therapy for ovulation induction (4). The Thessaloniki consensus provided normative protocols while planning ovulation induction in PCOS women and emphasized the negative role of obesity on expected outcomes (3). Again, there are also studies showing that metformin administration may increase the live birth and pregnancy rate in PCOS patients who receive gonadotropins for ovulation induction (5).

In general, none of the available studies include patients who are potentially responsive, and they exclude those potentially not responsive, such as those with obesity or other dysmetabolic conditions. I suggest that much more attention should be paid to defining responsiveness before any treatment is planned on an individual or categorical basis. Defining unresponsiveness ex-post can be useful on a scientific basis, but it does not fit with the individual needs of each individual patient. In a clinical background, each patient expects the most effective treatment based on his or her condition and his or her needs. In the following section focusing on "Obesity, Infertility, PCOS, and Weight Loss: Do We Need a More Personalized Approach?", I discuss some potential aspects that should be considered to finalize each treatment according to these concepts. For example, sustained weight loss could be very important before gonadotropin treatment for ovulation induction. Many more clinical studies are warranted in this area.

Diet Influences and Potential Effects on Infertility

A healthy diet may improve fertility for women with ovulatory dysfunction although data regarding the effects of variations in diet on fertility in anovulatory women, particularly those with PCOS, are few. Apart from lowering the malformation risk by periconceptional supplementation of folic acid, data on dietary integration with different micronutrients are often anecdotal. A potential efficacy of the Mediterranean dietary patterns has been emphasized in some studies. Other studies suggested that avoiding trans fats could also be of some help (6). Due to the potential benefit and low costs of a preconception diet, which still lacks powerful scientific evidence, much more research in this area and larger trials should be carried out, particularly before an ovulation induction protocol is planned.

Vitamin D levels are often lower than normal in obese PCOS women. The role of vitamin D in reproductive physiology has been investigated in the last year, and several studies have documented that supplementation with vitamin D may significantly improve ovulation in women with PCOS and be a possible benefit in patients undergoing ovulation induction techniques. Due to the potential benefit and low costs of a preconception diet, much more research in this area is warranted, particularly before an ovulation induction protocol is planned.

Specific interest has arisen on the potential role of advanced glycation end products (AGEs) in both the etiology of PCOS and related infertility. Once formed, AGEs may damage cellular structures via a number of mechanisms, after accumulation in various tissues, including the ovaries (7). Serum and tissue (including ovary) AGE levels depend on both endogenous and exogenous sources. Human and animal studies have shown that serum and tissue AGEs can be influenced by diet, particularly by methods of cooking, such as precooked fast food meals heated at high temperatures. Increased AGEs in women with PCOS have been found to be related to multiple metabolic derangements, insulin resistance, obesity, and inflammatory biomarkers. Reducing AGE intake may have potential implications in the treatment of infertile women with PCOS, offering specific dietary advice to improve not only their dysmetabolic milieu but also in improving their reproductive potential.

Obesity, Infertility, PCOS, and Weight Loss:
Do We Need a More Personalized Approach?

Because there is consistent evidence that raised body mass index (BMI) has adverse effects on ovulation induction treatment outcomes, women undergoing assisted reproduction may offer a unique opportunity to search for associations between preconceptional exposures and reproductive outcomes. In women with PCOS, obesity may favor the hyperandrogenic milieu and worsen the insulin-resistant state and metabolism. In addition, cytokine- and adipokine-related obesity and the associated low-grade inflammatory state may affect ovarian performance and favor anovulation. Obesity may affect oocyte quality and embryo growth because of lipotoxicity responses. Most of these factors may negatively impact the developmental competence of the oocytes, particularly in women with PCOS. This area of research promises to expand our knowledge on the impact of obesity in favoring infertility and in conditioning the efficacy of ovulation induction techniques.

Weight loss through lifestyle modification and bariatric surgery has been demonstrated to restore menstrual cyclicity. Accordingly, the British Fertility Society issued policy and practice guidelines advising clinicians to defer any treatment of obese women's BMI (8). Unfortunately, very few studies assessing clinical reproductive outcomes, quality of life, and treatment satisfaction in women with PCOS are available. In addition, although there are clinical recommendations of advising overweight or obese women to lose weight prior planning any ovulation induction technique, there is still some concern about the overall quality of the studies published on the topic. Finally, we still lack randomized controlled trials comparing dietary intervention to nonstructured dietary intervention.

The Relationship between Thyroid Dysfunction, Infertility, and Adverse Pregnancy Outcomes Needs to Be Further Investigated

A specific chapter of this book has been dedicated to thyroid dysfunctions and infertility. The association between hypothyroidism and infertility has been well known for a long period of time; however, in an endocrine setting, the incidence of infertility issues has often been considered a relatively uncommon event. The advent and worldwide explosion of ovulation induction techniques has led to some concerns about this association because lower implantation rates and increased rates of miscarriages have been associated with hypothyroidism. The exact prevalence of hypothyroidism among infertile women is still unknown and undoubtedly represents a challenge for future research. Although treatment of hypothyroidism with l-thyroxine has been found to potentially restore normal menses and improve fertility, prospective clinical trials designed according to well-defined objectives are nonetheless still lacking. On the other hand, preliminary studies in women with subclinical hypothyroidism undergoing ovulation induction techniques have also found significantly lowered miscarriages rates and higher delivery rates. Due to the large epidemiological relevance of hypothyroidism in women in reproductive age, this is undoubtedly an important area for further research in order to avoid excessive alarm and a consequent excessive request for health care and an increase in patient-paid costs.

Do Insulin Sensitizers Increase the Effectiveness of Clomiphene Citrate (CC) in the Treatment of Anovulatory Women with PCOS?

Treatment of infertility in women with PCOS may also include the insulin sensitizer metformin, combined or not with lifestyle intervention, as a potential pro-ovulatory agent. The use of metformin became widely used for a long period of time, particularly after studies showing that this drug was able to increase ovulation rates stimulated by a single cycle with CC in women with PCOS. In addition, the combination of metformin and lifestyle intervention appears to be another rationale choice for PCOS women with excess body weight although appropriate randomized controlled trials are warranted. At present, CC is considered as representing the first-line pharmacological therapy in PCOS women. As expected, a multicenter trial confirmed that CC is superior to metformin in inducing ovulation and in achieving better pregnancy outcomes, particularly live births (9). Nonetheless, these final results cannot be used to reject the potential benefit of metformin in selected PCOS patients. In fact, many studies other than that cited above support the concept that metformin, given for a long period of time, may add some significant effect to CC. This may be partly due to the fact that CC and metformin not only have different mechanisms of action but also different pharmacodynamics, which imply time-dependent effects on ovarian function. There are still several questions regarding the role of metformin in the treatment of infertile women with PCOS although it should be considered that the recent Guidelines by the Endocrine Society (10) recommend CC as the first-line treatment of anovulatory infertility in women with PCOS while suggesting the use of metformin as an adjuvant therapy for infertility to prevent OHSS in women with PCOS undergoing ovulation induction techniques. These suggestions may ultimately guide clinical practice worldwide until new data support the opportunity for an individualized use of metformin in infertile women with PCOS.

Inositols in the Treatment of Infertile PCOS: Is There a Role?

Based on available studies, the recent Endocrine Society Guidelines (10) recommended against the use of other insulin sensitizers, such as inositols, due to lack of benefit, for the treatment of PCOS. On the other hand, the use of inositols became very popular in the last years worldwide, so we have to take into consideration appropriate clinical trials in well-selected infertile PCOS women, aimed at achieving powerful data in favor or against the use of inositols.

Aromatase Inhibitors and Infertility in Women with PCOS: A New Challenge?

All clinicians involved in infertility, particularly in women with PCOS, are undoubtedly aware of the fact that CC has some intrinsic drawbacks related to the nonresponsiveness in many women with PCOS, some degree of resistance to ovulate, a relatively high rate of multiple pregnancies, and adverse side effects. Aromatase inhibitors, which centrally block the hypothalamic–pituitary–ovarian function, have been shown to favor fertility rates in otherwise infertile PCOS women. A recent double blind, multicenter, randomized trial tested the hypothesis that letrozole would be superior to CC as an infertility treatment and result in a better pregnancy outcomes (11). The main results in favor of letrozole were significantly increased cumulative ovulation rate and live births, no significant between-group differences in pregnancy loss, or more twin pregnancies. There is, however, still some concern about several aspects involving letrozole use in infertile PCOS women, which mainly relate to the following: (a) whether the efficacy is similar in obese versus normal weight women; (b) the opportunity to add a lifestyle intervention plan in obese PCOS women; (c) its likely inefficacy on androgens; (d) the lack of definition of a s.c. letrozole resistance, and, finally, (e) the fetal risk. In fact, some potential teratogenic and embryotoxic or fetotoxic activity has been reported animal models (12). Therefore, further research is undoubtedly warranted in this area.

A Future for Stem Cell Biology in the Treatment of Infertility?

Stem cell biology may represent an exciting future challenge for the treatment of reproductive disorders. Current research suggests that human ovaries contain stem cells that form new oocytes even in adulthood and that these stem cells can be cultured in vitro to develop into mature oocytes. Although we still have much to understand about stem cells, their potential applications in reproductive biology and medicine are countless.

Should Collaboration among Different Specializations Be Necessary to Improve Medical Treatment of Infertility?

At present, although the potential effectiveness of the treatment of women affected by infertility is difficult to define, a relatively small number of these women may still successfully deliver a baby, so how to define success represents a continuously changing challenge in spite of the continuous development of new technologies. As reported in a number of chapters in this book, obesity, insulin resistance, thyroid alterations, and other hormonal disturbances are potentially involved in favoring infertility in women at risk, particularly in PCOS patients. In addition, there is worldwide epidemiological evidence that subclinical hypothyroidism affects young or middle-aged women. For many women, professional collaboration between physicians directly involved in ovulation induction procedures and other specialists, particularly endocrinologists, psychologists, and internists could be very helpful in improving fertility rates.

Statements and Recommendations

- The use of AMH may represent a new biomarker of anovulatory amenorrhea, provided an international standard based on assays with high accuracy, precision, sensitivity, and reproducibility are available.

- A lifestyle approach should always be planned in anovulatory infertile women before planning an ovulation induction protocols; this is particularly relevant in women with excess weight or obesity.

- Infertile obese women, specifically those with PCOS, may achieve significant benefit even after modest (5%–10%) weight loss on ovulation rate and on their response to ovulation induction.

- Thyroid dysfunction should always be investigated and, if necessary, treated before starting ovulation induction.

- Collaboration among different specialists could considerably improve medical treatment of infertility in women, particularly those with PCOS.

REFERENCES

1. ESHRE Capri Workshop Group. Health and fertility in World Health Organization group 2 anovulatory women. Hum Reprod Update. 2012; 18:586–99.
2. Dewailly D, Andersen CY, Balen A, Broekmans F, Dilaver N, Fanchin R et al. The physiology and clinical utility of anti-Mullerian hormone in women. Hum Reprod Update. 2014; 20:370–85.
3. Thessaloniki ESHRE/ASRM-Sponsored PCOS Consensus Workshop Group. Consensus on infertility treatment related to polycystic ovary syndrome. Fertil Steril. 2008; 89:505–22.
4. Perales-Puchalt A, Legro RS. Ovulation induction in women with polycystic ovary syndrome. Steroids. 2013; 78:767–72.
5. Palomba S, Falbo A, La Sala GB. Metformin and gonadotropins for ovulation induction in patients with polycystic ovary syndrome: A systematic review with meta-analysis of randomized controlled trials. Reprod Biol Endocrinol. 2014 Jan 3; 12:3. doi: 10.1186/1477-7827-12-3
6. Vujkovic M, de Vries JH, Lindemans J, Macklon NS, van der Spek PJ, Steegers EA, Steegers-Theunissen RP. The preconception Mediterranean dietary pattern in couples undergoing in vitro fertilization/intracytoplasmic sperm injection treatment increases the chance of pregnancy. Fertil Steril. 2010; 94: 2096–101.
7. Merhi Z. Advanced glycation end products and their relevance in female reproduction. Hum Reprod. 2014; 135–45.
8. Balen AH, Anderson RA. Impact of obesity on female reproductive health: British Fertility Society, Policy and Practice Guidelines. Hum Fertil. 2007; 10:195–206.
9. Legro RS, Barnhart HX, Schlaff WD, Carr BR, Diamond MP, Carson SA et al. N Engl J Med. 2007; 356:551–66.
10. Legro RS, Arslanian SA, Ehrmann DA, Hoeger KM, Murad MH, Pasquali R, Welt CK. Endocrine Society diagnosis and treatment of polycystic ovary syndrome: An Endocrine Society clinical practice guideline. J Clin Endocrinol Metab. 2013; 98:4565–92.
11. Legro RS, Brzyski RG, Diamond MP, Coutifaris C, Schlaff WD, Casson P et al. Letrozole versus clomiphene for infertility in the polycystic ovary syndrome. N Engl J Med. 2014; 371:119–29.
12. Palomba S. Aromatase inhibitors for ovulation induction. J Clin Endocrinol Metab. 2015; 100:1742–7.

29

Summary: Levels of Evidence of Statements

Levels of Evidence Used in Statements

1a	Systematic review and meta-analysis of randomized controlled trials
1b	At least one randomized controlled trial
2a	At least one well-designed controlled study without randomization
2b	At least one other type of well-designed quasiexperimental study
3	Well-designed, nonexperimental descriptive studies, such as comparative studies, correlation studies, or case studies
4	Expert committee reports or opinions and/or clinical experience of respected authorities

TABLE 1.1

Level of Evidence of Statements

Statement	Level of Evidence
The initial growth of primordial follicles (also referred to as primary recruitment) is random, being independent of FSH. The cohort size of healthy early antral follicles recruited during the luteo-follicular transition is around 10 per ovary.	3
Inhibin A, secreted by maturing follicle and corpus luteum, has a direct endocrine role in the negative feedback on pituitary FSH production.	2b
Although the LH surge is believed to be the physiological signal for peri-ovulatory events, a mid-cycle bolus of FSH can replace LH and elicit oocyte maturation, ovulation, early luteinization of granulosa cells, and successful pregnancy.	2b
The major roles of E2 on uterine endometrium are for endometrial growth and for enabling P to act on the tissue.	2b
Kisspeptin and neurokinin B (NKB), neuropeptides secreted by the same neuronal population in the ventral hypothalamus, have emerged recently as critical central regulators of GnRH and thus gonadotropin secretion (5,6).	2b

TABLE 2.1

Level of Evidence of Statements

Statement	Level of Evidence
Chronic anovulation is a major cause of subfertility.	3
Chances for ovulation and pregnancy decrease when the duration of the menstrual cycle is prolonged.	3
Establishing the diagnosis of PCOS is complicated in adolescents and menopausal women.	4
Patients with less severe metabolic derangement will be added to the PCOS group using the Rotterdam criteria instead of the NIH criteria.	3

TABLE 3.1

Level of Evidence of Statements

Statement	Level of Evidence
WHO class 1 anovulation results from either congenital or acquired causes.	4
Based on the presence or absence of an olfaction defect, CHH is divided into two groups: CHH with anosmia/hyposmia and idiopathic CHH with normal olfaction.	4
Beside anosmia/hyposmia, Kallmann syndrome may include craniofacial, neurosensorial, and dysmorphic anomalies.	4
FHA represents 15% of cases of secondary amenorrhea and is the second leading cause of acquired HH after hyperprolactinemia.	4
FHA is a reversible form of GnRH deficiency due to a negative energy balance.	4
30%–50% of patients with FHA have polycystic ovarian morphology at ultrasound without real PCOS.	4

TABLE 4.1

Level of Evidence of Statements

Statement	Level of Evidence
Most anovulatory women with normal gonadotrophin and estradiol levels have PCOS.	3
Normogonadotropic normoestrogenic anovulation without PCOS may be caused by other endocrine disorders, for example, thyroid disease, hyperprolactinemia, pathology of the adrenal gland.	3
Long-term health consequences in women with normogonadotropic normoestrogenic anovulation but without PCOS are unknown.	4

TABLE 5.1

Level of Evidence of Statements

Statement	Level of Evidence
PCOS is diagnosed by two of these three criteria: hyperandrogenism, oligomenorrhea, or polycystic ovaries.	5
Oligomenorrhea and polycystic ovaries are common among adolescent women and confound the diagnosis in this age group.	2
Women with PCOS are at increased risk for infertility.	1a
Women with PCOS share many of the risk factors for endometrial cancer and may be at increased risk.	3a
Obesity is associated with increased metabolic risk and hyperandrogenism.	1a
Women with PCOS have an increased prevalence of anxiety and depression.	2a
Women with PCOS have an increased prevalence of cardiovascular risk factors, including family history of early cardiovascular disease, cigarette smoking, impaired glucose tolerance or type 2 diabetes, hypertension, dyslipidemia, obstructive sleep apnea, and obesity (especially increased abdominal adiposity).	2a
Despite the adverse cardiometabolic profile, there are not clear data supporting early onset or increase prevalence of cardiovascular events.	2c

TABLE 6.1

Level of Evidence of Statements

Statement	Level of Evidence
Alkylating agents induce POI in 40%–50% of women.	3
Chemotherapeutic agents damage the ovary by increasing follicle loss.	2b
The most common genetic cause of POI is chromosome X abnormalities.	2b
POF1 and POF2 regions located on Xq chromosome are necessary for ovarian follicle maintenance.	2a
POI is associated with familial or personal history of autoimmune diseases in 4%–5% of patients.	3
Premutation of *FRM1* gene is present in 13% of familial cases of POI.	2b
NOBOX mutation is present in 5%–7% of POI patients.	2b
More than 30 genes have been identified so far as candidate genes in human POI.	2b

TABLE 7.1

Level of Evidence of Statements

Statement	Level of Evidence
CAHs influence reproduction, either as the consequence of adrenal androgen excess or as the result of a severe deficiency in the synthesis and secretion of gonadal steroids.	2a
Patients with 3β-hydroxysteroid dehydrogenase, 17α-hydroxylase, and steroidogenic acute response protein/20-22 desmolase deficiencies present with female hypogonadism or male pseudohermaphroditism, and most are infertile.	3
The presentation of nonclassic CAH may be indistinguishable from functional forms of female hyperandrogenism.	2a
Infertility is common in classic CAH, and its severity parallels that of the enzymatic deficiency.	2a
Many women with classic CAH never try to conceive.	2a
Increased androgen concentrations and increased non-cycling progesterone levels in women and inhibition of gonadotropin secretion and testicular adrenal rest tumors in men may contribute to infertility.	2b
Intensification of replacement therapy in women with classic CAH results in pregnancy rates comparable to that of the normal population, yet the fertility rates are much lower.	2b
A significant number of women with classic CAH require ovulation induction or assisted reproductive technology to conceive.	2a
Fertility is not severely compromised in nonclassic CAH, and many patients conceive spontaneously.	2b
If glucocorticoid replacement is not useful in restoring ovulation in women with nonclassic CAH, clomiphene or gonadotropins can be used.	2b
Carrier frequencies for alleles causing classic 21α-hydroxylase deficiency are approximately 1:60, and the risk of a patient with classic 21α-hydroxylase deficiency of having a child with classic CAH is 1:20.	2a
Women with nonclassic 21α-hydroxylase deficiency may give birth to a fetus affected with classic 21α-hydroxylase deficiency because they frequently are compound heterozygotes for mild and severe mutations.	2b
Experimental prenatal treatment with exogenous dexamethasone may prevent virilization of affected female fetuses in approximately 80%–85% of cases.	2b
This treatment is currently being questioned because dexamethasone may have significant maternal and fetal side effects.	2a

TABLE 8.1

Level of Evidence of Statements

Statement	Level of Evidence
Thyroid dysfunction is associated with menstrual disturbances.	3
Treatment of thyroid dysfunction will restore menstrual cyclicity.	2b
Ovulation induction with clomiphene citrate and tamoxifen has uncertain effects on thyroid function.	4
Ovulation induction with gonadotrophins leads to a lowering in fT4 in women with thyroid autoimmunity.	1b

TABLE 9.1

Level of Evidence of Statements[a]

Statement	Level of Evidence
Dynamic testing to evaluate hyperprolactinemia should not be applied.	1b
A single prolactin assessment for the diagnosis of hyperprolactinemia is enough.	1b
Other causes of hyperprolactinemia should be excluded.	1a
Asymptomatic hyperprolactinemia does not need any treatment.	4
Microprolactinoma that only have irregular menses can be treated with oral contraceptives or cabergoline.	4
Cessation or switch of medication causes hyperprolactinemia.[b]	2b
Symptomatic micro- and macroadenomas should be treated with dopamine agonist.	1c
Cabergoline is the drug of choice because it has the highest efficacy in normalizing prolactin and tumor shrinkage.	1c
Women with prolactinomas need to discontinue dopamine agonist as soon as they know that they are pregnant.	3b
During pregnancy, prolactin assessment in prolactinoma patients is redundant.	1b
If dopamine agonists are indicated during pregnancy, bromocriptine is the drug of choice.	3a

[a] Summary of Endocrine Society Clinical Practice Guideline (13).

[b] Antipsychotic drugs should not be discontinued or switched without consent of the treating psychiatrist.

TABLE 11.1

Level of Evidence of Statements

Statement	Level of Evidence
Hypogonadotropic hypogonadism is characterized by low levels of FSH, and LH along with low levels of estradiol; it is classified as WHO class 1 anovulation.	2
In HH (WHO class 1) patients, anosmia or hyposmia is suggestive for Kallmann syndrome.	2
Normogonadotropic normo-estrogenic anovulation is characterized by normal levels of FSH, LH, and estradiol; it is classified as WHO class 2 anovulation. The majority of these women also suffer from polycystic ovary syndrome (PCOS).	2
PCOS should be diagnosed according to the Rotterdam consensus.	3
According to the Rotterdam consensus, the diagnosis of PCOS should be made if two of the three following criteria are met: androgen excess, ovulatory dysfunction, or polycystic ovarian morphology (PCOM).	2
A normal bleeding interval is between 21 and 35 days.	3
Hirsutism is defined as a Ferriman-Gallwey score of 8 or higher. Biochemical hyperandrogenism is defined as an elevated testosterone level or an elevated free androgen index (FAI) [T × 100/SHBG].	3
PCOM is defined as an increased number of follicles per ovary. The cutoff depends on the frequency of the transducer used. In case a FNPO is not assessable, ovarian volume might be used.	2
Cutoff values for clinical and biochemical hyperandrogenism are laboratory and age as well as ethnicity dependent.	2
Other causes of anovulation (thyroid disease or hyperpolactinemia) or HA (classical and non-classical forms of congenital adrenal hyperplasia, adrenal tumors, and Cushing's disease) should be ruled out before the diagnosis of PCOS can be made.	2
Hypergonadotropic hypogonadism is characterized by elevated levels of FSH and LH along with low levels of estradiol; it is classified as WHO class III anovulation. The monotropic rise in FSH is pathognomonic in these patients.	2
Patients with POI typically present with primary or secondary amenorrhea.	2
POI is often accompanied by complaints, such as hot flashes, night sweats, neurocognitive complaints as well as sexual problems such as loss of libido and dyspareunia.	2
Assessment of AMH levels or AFC measurements might aid the diagnosis of anovulatory infertility.	3

TABLE 12.1

Level of Evidence of Statements

Statement	Level of Evidence
Ovulation induction and controlled ovarian hyperstimulation are two different treatment options and should not be mixed up.	GPP
Controlled ovarian hyperstimulation in non-IVF should aim at achieving two to three follicles.	1a
COH-IUI should be a first-line treatment option in couples with mild male and unexplained subfertility when spontaneous chances of pregnancy are low.	1b
It remains unclear whether luteal support clearly improves cost-effectiveness of COH-IUI cycles.	1a

TABLE 13.1

Level of Evidence of Statements

Statement	Level of Evidence
There is insufficient evidence to define which monitoring methods are the most safe and cost-effective. US monitoring is the most advisable method for monitoring in OI.	4
The pregnancy-related diameter of the leading follicle in CC cycles varies between 18 and 22 mm.	3
The pregnancy-related diameter of the leading follicle in gonadotropin cycles varies between 17 and 21 mm.	3
There is insufficient evidence about a pregnancy related cutoff point for endometrium thickness in OI cycles.	3
There is insufficient evidence that US monitoring in CC cycles improves pregnancy rates. There is no sufficient evidence to suggest that US monitoring in CC cycles reduces multiple pregnancy rates.	1a
US monitoring in gonadotropin cycles is mandatory.	4

TABLE 14.1

Level of Evidence for Statements

Statement	Level of Evidence
One relatively small comparative nonrandomized study showed a nonsignificant higher cumulative conception rate with the pulsatile GnRH and a nonsignificantly lower rate of multiple pregnancies.	3
Case studies show ovulation rate/cycle of 70%–100% and 38%–97% with pulsatile GnRH and gonadotropins, respectively.	3
Case studies show pregnancy rates/cycle of 9%–30% and 20%–93% with pulsatile GnRH and gonadotropins, respectively.	3
Case studies show multiple pregnancy rates of 0%–17% and 15%–38% with pulsatile GnRH and gonadotropins, respectively.	3
Pulsatile GnRH does not require hormonal luteal support treatment.	4
Pulsatile GnRH treatment requires simple once-a-month monitoring for verification of ovulation, resulting in less burden for the patient.	4
Ovarian hyperstimulation is a very rare if not absent side effect of pulsatile GnRH treatment.	4
Most reported side effect is local inflammation at injection site.	4

TABLE 15.1

Level of Evidence for Statements

Statement	Level of Evidence
CC used for hypothalamic–pituitary dysfunction—WHO Group 2, mainly PCOS, increases ovulation and pregnancy rates compared with placebo.	1a
Clomiphene plus dexamethasone treatment is effective in increasing pregnancy rate compared to clomiphene alone.	1a
The routine addition of hCG in a CC cycle does not improve conception rates.	1a
CC is superior to metformin in achieving live birth in infertile women with PCOS.	1b
Letrozole produces higher live birth and pregnancy rates in subfertile women with anovulatory PCOS, compared to CC.	1a
No evidence of a difference in effect was found between clomiphene versus tamoxifen.	1a
Pregnancies and live births are achieved more effectively and faster after low-dose FSH versus CC for first-line treatment.	1b
There is no convincing evidence of an increase in the risk of ovarian tumors following CC treatment.	1a

TABLE 16.1

Level of Evidence of Statements

Statement	Level of Evidence
Ovulation induction for PCOS patients with letrozole compared to clomiphene citrate (followed by timed intercourse) results in a significantly higher live birth rate for letrozole treatment.	1a
In a clomiphene citrate–resistant PCOS population, letrozole results in a comparable live birth rate to ovarian drilling.	1a
After a clomiphene failure in more than one cycle, for the purpose of ovulation induction, pregnancy rates are equivalent for letrozole versus gonadotropin injections.	1b
Higher pregnancy rates are achieved when the leading follicles are in the 23 to 28 mm range for letrozole ovulation induction cycles.	3
Compared to timed intercourse, IUI does not seem to increase the pregnancy rate in couples with PCOS and normal semen analysis treated with letrozole for ovulation induction.	3
Vaginal progesterone luteal support after letrozole ovulation induction may result in a higher clinical pregnancy rate in women with PCOS.	3

TABLE 17.1

Level of Evidence for Statements

Statement	Level of Evidence
Metformin should not be first-line therapy for ovulation induction and should not be commenced until intensive lifestyle modification has been attempted.	1b

TABLE 18.1

Level of Evidence of Statements

Statement	Level of Evidence
LEO is not superior to CC as a first-line treatment in anovulatory PCOS women.	1b
LEO and gonadotrophins are equally effective in inducing ovulation and generating pregnancies in CC-resistant PCOS women.	1a
LEO is associated with lower risks of multiple pregnancy compared to gonadotrophins.	1a
Four punctures (7–8 mm deep) per ovary with a power setting of 30–40 watts for 5 seconds per puncture seem to be the optimum dose of monopolar ovarian electrocautery.	2
Approximately, 50% of PCOS women continue to benefit from LEO for many years.	2
Both bipolar and monopolar techniques of LEO have proven long-term safety.	2

TABLE 19.1

Level of Evidence of Statements

Statement	Level of Evidence
In women with WHO 2 anovulation as the main cause of infertility, the use of step-up protocols significantly reduces the risk of multiple pregnancies.	1a
The starting dose of gonadotropins and the risk of over-response can be assessed by prediction models.	1a
A frequent monitoring every 5–7 days using ultrasound assessment and hormonal determination is able to prevent the risk of over-response.	1b
The safety of low-dose and chronic low-dose protocols is higher than the conventional one.	1b
Small FSH dose increments of 50% of the initial or previous FSH dose are less likely to result in excessive stimulation.	1b
When more than three growing follicles are observed on ultrasound in young women, the risk of multiple pregnancies is increased.	1b
The concomitant use of a GnRH agonist and gonadotropins does not improve pregnancy rates and is associated with an increased risk of OHSS.	1a
The introduction of GnRH antagonist during stimulation for WHO 2 anovulation is not absolutely required except in presence of premature progesterone elevation.	1b

TABLE 20.1

Level of Evidence of Statements

Statement	Level of Evidence
Modest weight loss achieved by lifestyle modification in overweight/obese women with WHO 2 anovulation contributes to resumption of ovulation.	2a
Limiting weight gain in women who are overweight or obese by means of lifestyle modification during pregnancy improves obstetric outcomes.	1a
Lifestyle modification for weight loss should include a healthy diet (reduced calorie intake) and increased exercise in combination with behavior modification.	1a

TABLE 21.1

Level of Evidence of Statements

Statement	Level of Evidence
Ovulation rates can reach up to 42% following ovulation induction.	1b
GnRH agonist pretreatment does not improve the results of ovulation induction.	1b
Estrogen therapy increased ovulation rate in a randomized trial, but this result is contradicted by smaller studies with a lower evidence level.	1b
Corticosteroid treatment may improve ovulation or pregnancy rates, but further research is required to substantiate this conclusion.	1b
Dehydroepiandrosterone does not improve the chances of ovulation or endocrine conditions in the ovary.	1b
Oocyte donation is more effective than ovulation induction for achieving pregnancy, but pregnancies following ovulation induction are more at risk for complications.	3

TABLE 22.1

Level of Evidence of Statements

Statement	Level of Evidence
Success of ovulation induction has multiple dimensions and depends on the stage and strategy of treatment.	2a
For cost-effectiveness analysis, fertility treatments are more difficult than for other types of medical care.	4
The definition of success of ovulation induction in clinical research can differ from the definition of success in daily practice.	4

TABLE 23.1

Level of Evidence of Statements

Statement	Level of Evidence
The purpose of ovulation induction is monofollicular growth and ovulation.	3
Multiple follicular development is associated with increased chances of (multiple) pregnancy.	1a
During ovulation induction, the chance of multiple follicle development is reduced by frequent monitoring and strict cancellation criteria.	3/4
Ultrasound as well as serum estradiol measurement can be utilized for monitoring follicle development during ovulation induction.	3
Low-dose gonadotropin protocols in ovulation induction decrease risk of multiple follicle development.	3
It is more difficult to accomplish monofollicular development in a patient with a more explicit PCOS phenotype.	3
Changes in endocrine milieu can decrease chances of multiple follicle development in ovulation induction.	1b
Using frequent monitoring and strict cancellation criteria during a low-dose step-up gonadotropin stimulation protocol results in 70%–80% monofollicular development.	3

TABLE 24.1

Level of Evidence of Statements

Statement	Level of Evidence
OHSS with ovulation induction is a rare complication.	2b
Women with PCOS or previous OHSS can be identified as women at risk of developing OHSS with ovulation induction.	4
Prevent OHSS by using a step-up protocol for ovulation induction with gonodotrophin.	2b
u-hCG versus rec-hCG trigger does not increase OHSS for ovulation induction combined with IUI.	2a
Trigger with GnRH analog reduced OHSS compared to hCG.	2a
HES 6% infusion during the time of IUI when ultrasound free fluid is present can prevent OHSS symptoms.	4
Rescue IVF is a valid option in case of over-response to prevent the development of OHSS.	3
Dopamine agonists might be useful for reducing OHSS symptoms, but the evidence is limited.	2b

TABLE 25.1

Level of Evidence of Statements

Statement	Level of Evidence
Pregnancy is more likely to occur with two follicles than with one in COS cycles (9).	1a
The risk of multiple pregnancies for two follicles as compared to one follicle increases by 6% (9).	1a
There is no difference in the risk of multiple pregnancies between anti-estrogens and gonadotropins in IUI programs (11).	1a

TABLE 26.1

Level of Evidence of Statements

Statement	Level of Evidence
Long-lasting underexposure to estrogens may lead, in these circumstances, to osteoporosis (i.e., decreased bone mineral density [BMD]), mood and cognitive disturbances, and sexual dysfunction as well as accelerated cardiovascular aging and subsequent cardiovascular disease and, if left untreated, a reduced life span.	2
WHO 2 anovulation and especially PCOS are associated with obesity, insulin resistance, and metabolic syndrome; these women also have an increased risk to develop type 2 diabetes, hypertension, and probably cardiovascular disease.	2
WHO 1 anovulation is associated with osteopenia, osteoporosis, endothelial dysfunction, and dyslipidemia compared to healthy ovulatory women.	2
Women with HH present with significantly higher depression and anxiety and also sexual problems compared to healthy subjects.	2
HH women have lowered PBM because of their hypo-estrogenic state along with other factors, such as low calcium and vitamin D3 intake, undernutrition, and excessive exercise.	2
HH is associated with significant coronary artery disease and endothelial dysfunction.	2
WHO 1 patients present a particular susceptibility to common life events, restrictive disordered eating, depressive traits, and psychosomatic disorders.	2
Increased adiposity, particularly abdominal, is associated with HA and increased metabolic risk.	
Women with PCOS are at an increased risk for developing impaired glucose tolerance and type 2 diabetes.	2
Weight loss is likely beneficial for both reproductive and metabolic dysfunction in this setting. Weight loss is likely insufficient as a treatment for PCOS in normal-weight women.	2
Women with PCOS suffer more often from psychological and behavioral disorders and reduced quality of life.	2
Women with PCOS share many of the risk factors associated with the development of endometrial cancer, including obesity, hyperinsulinism, type 2 diabetes, and abnormal uterine bleeding. Hence, they do have an increased lifelong risk for developing endometrial cancer.	2
Early menopause has been associated with increased CVD risk.	2
Women with early menopause are at higher risk of angina after myocardial infarction (MI), independent of comorbidities, severity and quality of care.	2
Bilateral oophorectomy leads to an increase in CVD as well as to an increase in neurological or mental diseases.	2
Women with POI experience more sexual dysfunction compared to healthy controls.	2
Women with POI are at risk for cognitive impairment.	2
Life expectancy in POI is about 2 years less than those who have menopause over 55 years, and this is thought to be due to an excess of deaths due to CVD, osteoporosis, and neurocognitive decline.	2
Nonhormonal therapies, such as SSRIs, serotonin and norepinephrine reuptake inhibitors, or gabapentin may have a role in the management of vasomotor symptoms in women who decline HRT or in whom HRT is contraindicated.	3
There is no evidence for the use of complementary or herbal preparations in POI.	2

TABLE 27.1

Level of Evidence of Statements

Statement	Level of Evidence
Body mass index and hyperandrogenemia seem the predominant predictors for ovulation after CC treatment.	2a
Age and cycle history seem the predominant predictors pregnancy rate after CC treatment.	2a
Metformin might be effective as an adjuvant to CC in CRA patients.	2a
Patients with hyperandrogenism (T and FAI) and elevated BMI had decreased chances of conceive after LEO.	2a
Presence of the FSH receptor polymorphism might predict clomiphene resistance.	2a

30

Summary: Grade of Strength of Recommendations

Grade of Strength of Evidence Used in Recommendations (Guidelines)

A	Directly based on Level 1 evidence
B	Directly based on Level 2 evidence or extrapolated recommendation from Level 1 evidence
C	Directly based on Level 3 evidence or extrapolated recommendation from either Levels 1 or 2 evidence
D	Directly based on Level 4 evidence or extrapolated recommendation from either Levels 1, 2, or 3 evidence
GPP	Good practice point (GPP)

TABLE 2.2

Grade of Strength for Recommendations

Recommendation	Grade Strength
WHO criteria should be used for classification of anovulation.	GPP
Diagnosing PCOS should be performed by using the Rotterdam criteria.	GPP

TABLE 3.2

Grade of Strength for Recommendations

Recommendation	Grade Strength
In CHH, it is important to evaluate all pituitary functions to eliminate an anterior hypopituitarism.	D
The genetic study is often the last step in the investigation of the CHH.	D
Although widely used, the diagnostic value of the GnRH test in CHH has been questioned because of its low profitability.	D
Hypothalamic/pituitary MRI must be performed systematically in FHA.	GPP
A psychiatric evaluation can be helpful for diagnosing an eating disorder.	GPP
The baseline serum LH assay can help differentiate FHA from PCOS.	GPP

TABLE 4.2

Grade of Strength for Recommendations

Recommendation	Grade Strength
In normogonadotropic anovulatory women, the presence of PCOS should be excluded.	GPP
After exclusion of PCOS, the presence of endocrinological disorders should be excluded by history-taking, pelvic ultrasound, and endocrine screening.	GPP

TABLE 5.2

Grade of Strength for Recommendations

Recommendation	Grade Strength
Other mimics, such as thyroid disease, prolactin excess, and congenital adrenal hyperplasia (21-hydroxylase deficiency), should be routinely excluded.	B
Rare causes of similar symptoms, such as Cushing's syndrome, androgen secreting tumor, or steroid abuse, should be selectively excluded.	B
Women with PCOS should not undergo routine screening with ultrasound or biopsy for endometrial cancer.	C
Women with PCOS should undergo routine screening for dysglycemia with an oral glucose tolerance test or a glycohemoglobin level.	A
Women with PCOS should undergo routine screening with a fasting lipid profile.	A
Women with PCOS should be selectively screened for sleep disorders and liver disease.	C
Other infertility factors should be considered in couples presenting with infertility presumed secondary to female PCOS-related anovulation.	A

TABLE 6.2

Grade of Strength for Recommendations

Recommendation	Grade Strength
In all patients, when POI is suspected, FSH should be measured twice, at least 1 month apart.	B
In all patients with POI, a karyotype should be performed.	B
In all patients with POI, an autoimmune cause of the disease should be ruled out.	B
TSH, anti-thyroid, and anti 21 hydroxylase antibodies should be measured.	B
In all patients with POI, premutation of *FMR1* gene should be searched for.	B
In all patients with POI, AMH serum level should be measured.	B
In patients with POI, NGS sequencing is able to test a panel of candidate genes.	B
Reversibility of POI is present in 4%–8% of POI women.	C
Hormone replacement therapy is necessary at least up to the age of natural menopause.	B

TABLE 7.2

Grade of Strength for Recommendations

Recommendation	Grade Strength
Nonclassic forms of 21α-hydroxylase and 11β-hydroxylase deficiencies are indistinguishable from other forms of class II oligoovulation and must be ruled out in certain populations because they carry a significant risk for having a child affected by classic CAH.	B
Patients with classic CAH seeking fertility usually require intensification of their adrenal steroid replacement therapy with the aim of suppressing androgen and progesterone excess and reducing testicular rest tumors in men.	B
Glucocorticoid replacement should be offered to women with nonclassic CAH trying to conceive.	B
Genetic counseling should be offered to patients with classic and nonclassic CAH.	B
Fetal sex determination by detection of the Y chromosome in males in the maternal serum (SRY test) may be useful to avoid prenatal dexamethasone in males.	C
Assisted reproductive technology permits preimplantation genetic diagnosis and avoidance of the transfer of affected embryos resulting from IVF.	D

TABLE 8.2

Grade of Strength for Recommendations

Recommendation	Grade Strength
Overt hypothyroidism and overt thyrotoxicosis should be treated in women desiring to become pregnant.	D
Subclinical hypothyroidism should be treated in women desiring to become pregnant with the aim of a TSH below 2.5 mU/L.	B

TABLE 9.2

Grade of Strength for Recommendations

Recommendation	Grade Strength
Macro-prolactin assessment is not useful in symptomatic individuals.	A
Usually, a single prolactin assessment will diagnose hyperprolactinemia.	A
Other causes of hyperprolactinemia should be excluded when a hyperprolactinemia diagnosis is established.	A
Symptomatic micro- or macroprolactinoma should be treated with a dopamine agonist.	A
Asymptomatic microprolactinoma do not need treatment.	C
In collaboration with an endocrinologist; formal visual field assessment followed by MRI without gadolinium in pregnant women with prolactinomas that experience severe headaches with or without visual field changes.	B

TABLE 11.2

Grade of Strength for Recommendations

Recommendation	Grade Strength
In anovulatory patients, FSH, LH, and estradiol should be determined during the initial workup. To rule out other pathologies, prolactin, TSH, and early morning cortisol should be measured too.	B
In anovulatory patients, a thorough history should be taken focusing on lifestyle habits (extreme exercise, poor caloric intake, and obesity), signs of other endocrinopathies (i.e., hypothalamic or pituitary lesions, hyperprolactinemia, hypothyroidism, and hyperthyroidism). The screening history should also focus on a family history of irregular cycles, HA, or early menopause along with a family history of autoimmune disorders (e.g., thyroid disorders, diabetes, Addison's disease, vitiligo, systemic lupus, rheumatoid arthritis, celiac disease), fragile X syndrome, or intellectual disability.	B
The physical examination should focus on body habitus, evidence of normal secondary sexual characteristics, hirsutism, and alopecia as well as evidence of vaginal atrophy secondary to hypo-estrogenism.	B
MRI might aid in the diagnosis of Kallmann syndrome and is mandatory in cases with multiple endocrinopathies to rule out tumors in the pituitary or midbrain regions.	B
Gn-RH testing is not cost-effective and not recommended. IGF-1 measurements are only recommended in WHO 1 patients without any sigs of pubertal development.	C
Accurate olfactory phenotyping in IHH subjects can inform the pathophysiology of this condition and guide genetic testing.	C
Renal ultrasound examination is recommended to patients with syndromic IHH, such as Kallmann syndrome, independent of the genetic basis.	C
Bone mineral density of the lumbar spine, femoral neck, and hip is recommended at the initial diagnosis of HH and after 1 to 2 years of sex steroid therapy in hypogonadal patients with osteoporosis or low trauma fracture.	C
PCOS should be diagnosed according to the Rotterdam consensus.	B
Clinical hyperandrogenism (HA) should be assessed using the Ferriman-Gallwey score. Biochemical HA should preferably be assessed according to the available assay (either LCM/S or RIA assays).	B
Adolescent PCOS is diagnosed if all three Rotterdam consensus characteristics of PCOS are present.	C
In postmenopausal women, the diagnosis is impossible to make but should be considered in women with a clear-cut history of irregular menstrual periods and signs of hyperandrogenism, such as hirsutism.	C
The diagnosis should be confirmed by obtaining two consecutive FSH measurements revealing levels in the menopausal range (>40 IU/L) at least 1 month apart in the setting of 6 months of amenorrhea.	B
Women with POI should be screened for X chromosome aberrations and for FMR1 gene (pre) mutations.	B
Women with POI should also be screened for auto-antibodies against adrenal, thyroid tissue, and thyroid stimulating hormone receptors and ovarian tissue.	B
Measurement of AMH or AFC is not routinely recommended for women with POI.	C
BMD measurements are not recommended in women with POI who have been treated with HRT since the time of diagnosis.	B

TABLE 12.2

Grade of Strength for Recommendations

Recommendation	Grade Strength
In couples with mild male or unexplained subfertility, COH-IUI should be a first-line treatment option when spontaneous chances are low.	A
Ovulation induction should result in mono-ovulation, COH in multi-ovulation (two or three dominant follicles).	GPP and A
Luteal support in COH-IUI should only be applied when proven cost-effective.	A

TABLE 13.2

Grade of Strength for Recommendations

Recommendation	Grade Strength
Vaginal US to monitor follicular growth during ovulation induction is advisable at least in the first treatment cycle when anti-estrogens are used, but it is considered mandatory in all gonadotropin cycles.	GPP
There is no sufficient evidence that US monitoring in CC cycles improves pregnancy rates. There is no sufficient evidence to suggest that US monitoring in CC cycles reduces multiple pregnancy rates.	A
Ovulation induction should only be initiated if patient and physician are prepared to cancel cycles with hyper-response in order to prevent OHSS and multiple pregnancies.	GPP
The pregnancy-related diameter in CC cycles is optimal when the leading follicle reaches 18–22 mm and in gonadotropin cycles when the leading follicle reaches 17–21 mm.	C
In order to avoid multiple pregnancy, achieving mono-follicular or maximal double follicular ovulation is advisable.	GPP
Specific cancellation criteria to prevent multiple pregnancies are recommended, such as no more than two follicles $\geqslant$14 mm, with the largest >17 mm and E_2 concentrations <600–1000 pg/ml.	D
Mid-luteal serum progesterone (P_4) measurement and urinary LH tests are well-established methods to detect ovulation in OI treatment.	D

TABLE 14.2

Grade of Strength for Recommendations

Recommendation	Grade Strength
Treatment with pulsatile GnRH is first choice treatment for ovulation induction for patients with WHO 1 patients with anovulation of supra-pituitary origin.	C/D
Starting dose should be 5 µg per 120 minutes subcutaneously during the first month or first cycle for prevention of multiple pregnancies.	C/D
Standard dose is otherwise 10 µg per 90 minutes.	D
Monitoring requires a once-a-month visit only for verification of ovulation by established means (BBT, mid-luteal progesterone, or ultrasound).	D
When adequate facilities are not available for pulsatile GnRH treatment, patients should be referred.	D
There is urgent need to conduct an adequate randomized controlled cost-effectiveness trial.	D

TABLE 15.2

Grade of Strength for Recommendations

Recommendation	Grade Strength
CC should be used as first-line treatment to induce ovulation in hypothalamic–pituitary dysfunction—WHO Group 2 women.	A
Even though the addition of dexamethasone as an adjunct to clomiphene therapy increases pregnancy rate, due to its side effects, it should probably be reserved for women who have an adrenal component as a cause for their anovulation.	D
If an anti-estrogen effect on endometrium appears with CC, other treatment options should be considered.	B
The preference of letrozole over CC as first-line treatment in anovulatory PCOS is encouraging (but letrozole is still not licensed for ovulation induction).	A

TABLE 16.2

Grade of Strength for Recommendations

Recommendation	Grade Strength
Letrozole is the treatment of choice for ovulation induction in PCOS patients (but letrozole is still not licensed for ovulation induction).	A
Letrozole is the treatment of choice in cases of clomiphene resistance or clomiphene failure.	A

TABLE 17.2

Grade of Strength for Recommendations

Recommendation	Grade Strength
Pharmacological ovulation induction should not be recommended for first-line therapy in women with polycystic ovary syndrome who are morbidly obese (body mass index ≥ 35 kg/m^2) until appropriate weight loss has occurred either through diet, exercise, bariatric surgery, or other appropriate means.	C
Metformin could be used alone to improve ovulation rate and pregnancy rate in women with polycystic ovary syndrome who are anovulatory, have a body mass index ≤ 30 kg/m^2, and are infertile with no other infertility factors.	B
If one is considering using metformin alone to treat women with polycystic ovary syndrome who are anovulatory, have a body mass index ≥ 30 kg/m^2, and are infertile with no other infertility factors, clomiphene citrate should be added to improve fertility outcomes.	A
Metformin should be combined with clomiphene citrate to improve fertility outcomes rather than persisting with further treatment with clomiphene citrate alone in women with polycystic ovary syndrome who are clomiphene citrate resistant, anovulatory, and infertile with no other infertility factors.	A

TABLE 18.2

Grade of Strength for Recommendations

Recommendation	Grade Strength
LEO cannot be recommended as a first-line treatment in anovulatory PCOS women.	A
Clomiphene citrate–resistant PCOS women should make an informed choice between LEO and gonadotrophin therapy, which are equally effective with possible advantages of LEO.	A
When using monopolar electrocautery, four punctures (7–8 mm deep) should be made into the anti-mesentric side of each ovary with a power setting of 30 watts for 5 seconds per puncture with minimal or no thermal damage to the ovarian surface.	B
LEO may be recommended in gonadotrophin-over-respondent PCOS women.	B

TABLE 19.2

Grade of Strength for Recommendations

Recommendation	Grade Strength
Although sometimes difficult to achieve, the goal of gonadotropin treatment is to promote the growth and development of a single mature follicle.	A
The starting dose of gonadotropin needs to be adjusted according to the patient's BMI: 37.5 to 75 IU/day in non-obese women, 75 to 112.5 IU in obese women.	A
Adherence to a 14-day starting period at least for the first cycle is less likely to result in excessive stimulation.	A
The dose increments should not exceed 50% of the preceding dose.	A
After six ovulatory cycles using gonadotropins, strategy needs to be reconsidered with the couple.	B
Low-dose FSH protocols are effective in achieving ovulation in women with WHO 2 anovulation, but further refinement is needed to better control the safety of these regimens.	A
Intense ovarian response monitoring is required to reduce complications and secure efficiency.	A
Strict cycle cancellation criteria should be agreed upon with the patient before therapy is started.	A
Preventing all multiple pregnancies and OHSS is not possible at this time.	A

TABLE 20.2

Grade of Strength for Recommendations

Recommendation	Grade Strength
Lifestyle modification targeting weight loss in overweight/obese women with WHO 2 anovulation and prevention of weight gain in lean women should be recommended for improving general health and well-being.	B
Preconception weight loss in overweight/obese women and limiting weight gain during pregnancy should be advised with the aim to decrease obesity-related pregnancy complications.	C
Lifestyle modification targeting weight loss in overweight/obese women with WHO 2 anovulation and prevention of weight gain in lean women should entail the combination of reduced calorie intake and increased exercise in combination with behavior modification.	C
Lifestyle modification for weight loss in overweight/obese women with WHO 2 anovulation and prevention of weight gain in lean women should entail face-to-face dietary advice and education on healthy food choices (irrespective of macronutrient composition) and instructions on increased exercise accompanied by behavior change techniques, personal guidance, and support.	D

TABLE 21.2

Grade of Strength for Recommendations

Recommendation	Grade Strength
Patients with POI should be informed about the low probability of achieving pregnancy spontaneously or through ovulation induction.	B
When opting for ovulation induction, treatment schemes should be individualized due to lacking and contradicting existing evidence.	B
When considering oocyte donation, patients should be counseled about the increased risk of pregnancy complications.	C

TABLE 22.2

Grade of Strength for Recommendations

Recommendation	Grade Strength
Studies should report on multiple cycles on the outcomes of ovulation and ongoing pregnancy.	B
Couples should be well informed on treatment effect on the cycle level and on the reproductive life of the woman and her family.	C
Side effects at all time points should be considered.	C
Cost-effectiveness of ovulation induction might be patient-tailored, involving different prognostic factors.	D
After counseling of the couple, shared decision making is recommended.	D

TABLE 23.2

Grade of Strength for Recommendations

Recommendation	Grade Strength
The aim of ovulation induction is monofollicular development.	C
Frequent monitoring and strict cancellation criteria are mandatory to prevent multiple follicle development.	B
A low-dose gonadotropin stimulation protocol should be used instead of a high-dose protocol, to reduce the complication risk.	B
The patient should be counseled about the multiple pregnancy risk before treatment starts.	D

TABLE 24.2

Grade of Strength for Recommendations

Recommendation	Grade Strength
Consider ovarian drilling for POCS patients.	D
Prophylactic LMWH in case of OHSS.	GPP
Secondary prevention involves cycle cancellation with or without GnRH antagonist treatment and cabergoline.	D
In over-response, use an GnHR agonist trigger and convert to IVF with freeze-all embryos.	D

TABLE 25.2

Grade of Strength for Recommendations

Recommendation	Grade Strength
Low-dose gonadotropins should be used instead of high-dose gonadotropins.	A
COS should aim for no more than two follicles.	B
Follicle aspiration may prevent multiple pregnancies while maintaining acceptable pregnancy rates.	C
In case of multifollicular development, escape ART (conversion from IUI into ART) can prevent multiple pregnancies while maintaining acceptable pregnancy rates when combined with single embryo transfer.	C

TABLE 26.2

Grade of Strength for Recommendations

Recommendation	Grade Strength
In WHO 1 HH women, more attention should be paid to exercise among women. For most of the young women, exercise causes a positive effect, improving health and physical fitness.	B
Especially the issue of the long-term consequences of HH on CVD risk needs to be cleared to possibly minimize the risk of cardiovascular events in this group of women.	C
Screening in adolescents and women with PCOS for increased adiposity, by BMI calculation and measurement of waist circumference, should be done routinely.	B
An oral glucose tolerance test (OGTT) (consisting of fasting and 2-hour glucose level using a 75-g oral glucose load) should be used to screen for impaired glucose tolerance (IGT) and T2DM in adolescents and adult women with PCOS.	B
Adolescents and women with PCOS should be screened for CVD risk factors, such as a family history of early CVD, cigarette smoking, IGT/T2DM, hypertension, dyslipidemia, obstructive sleep apnea, and obesity (especially increased abdominal adiposity).	B
Exercise therapy in the management of overweight and obesity in PCOS might be helpful.	C
Weight loss strategies should start with calorie-restricted diets (with no evidence that one type of diet is superior) for adolescents and women with PCOS who are overweight or obese.	C
The use of hormonal contraceptives (i.e., oral contraceptives, patch, or vaginal ring) as first-line management for menstrual abnormalities is recommended. Especially in case hirsutism or acne is part of PCOS, this approach treats both entities.	B
Screen women and adolescents with PCOS for depression and anxiety by history and, if identified, providing appropriate referral and/or treatment.	B
Routine ultrasound screening for endometrial thickness in women with PCOS should not be done.	B
Women with POI should be treated with HRT to reduce their complaints as well as their risk for CVD.	C
Women with POI and sexual dysfunction should be counseled by a sexologist and treated with HRT.	C
Women with cognitive impairment due to POI seem to benefit from HRT.	C
HRT has not been successful in reversing the effects of reproductive aging to prevent long-term morbidity and mortality.	B
General lifestyle and dietary measures to reduce risk of cardiovascular disease (CVD) and osteoporosis should be recommended.	B
Do not use bisphosphonates in women who are trying to establish a pregnancy.	B

TABLE 27.2

Grade of Strength for Recommendations

Recommendation	Grade Strength
Body mass index and hyperandrogenemia seem the predominant predictors for ovulation induction outcome.	B
Individual patient characteristics should be taken into account.	D
Prognostic models can be supportive in terms of clinical decision making.	D

Index

This index includes the Foreword. Page numbers with f, t, and r refer to figures, tables, and references, respectively.

Milton Keynes UK
Ingram Content Group UK Ltd.
UKHW051934141024
449569UK00027B/1488